OBTAIN KEYS TO SLOW THE AGING PROCESS

LEARN HOW NUTRITION CAN INCREASE LONGEVITY

FIND OUT WHAT POLITICS AND PATIENTS HAVE IN COMMON

LEARN WHAT TO AVOID IN THE FOOD, MANUFACTURING, MEDICAL AND PHARMACEUTICAL INDUSTRIES

DISCOVER HOW AND WHY GOD'S "FOOD" IS THE ULTIMATE SOURCE OF HEALTH

YOU WILL BE ENCOURAGED TO DEMAND MEDICAL FREEDOM OF CHOICE

HEALTH

IN THE 21ST CENTURY

Will Doctors Survive?

FRANCISCO CONTRERAS MD

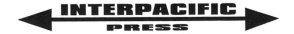

Chula Vista, Calif.

Published by
INTERPACIFIC PRESS
PO BOX 7597
CHULA VISTA, CA 91912
Telephone: (619) 428-0930
Toll Free: (800) 950-6505
Fax: (619) 428-0994

Printed by
BookCrafters

First Printing: February 1997

Cover Design by Jack Hanley, Alex Phillips, Felipe Contreras
Editors: Pamela Lowe, Carmen & Michael Wood,
Daniel E. Kennedy
Spanish Edition Editor: Luisa Ruiz

■ ISBN 1-57946-000-3
Library of Congress Card. No. 97-70184

DEDICATION

To my father, Dr. Ernesto Contreras Sr., who has lived up to
the true principles of medicine, placing his patients' concerns
above all. Conscious of the consequences of fighting against
the establishment, he made every sacrifice necessary to offer
alternative choices where there was none.

And to my mother, Rita Contreras, for her material and emotional commitment, for motivating her children to be sup-
portive as a family and for sharing with my father the power
of one mission: to heal bodies and souls.

ACKNOWLEDGMENTS

This book would not have been accomplished without the expertise of Luisa Ruiz. She braved the difficult and tedious task of organizing all the research, and her encouragement and guidance in the art of writing was the force that pulled it all together. Preparing the English version was a monumental task. Michael Wood, Carmen Wood and Dr. Howard Conrad not only translated most of the book, but they helped me "culturalize" the information for the American and other English-speaking readers. The editorial work by Pam Lowe and Dr. Mary Ruth Swope were invaluable.

The constructive input of Daniel E. Kennedy elevated the quality of the way the information is presented. Daniel's commitment to this book has been a powerful moral and spiritual support. The immeasurable enthusiasm of Jack Hanley is the driving force behind this project, and his expertise has greatly enriched my life. How he kept track of the million details of generating and publishing this book, I will never know.

Israel Arana, our computer wizard, formatted the book, and composed all the graphics. The artwork by Alex Phillips and Felipe Contreras was excellent. I thank the Oasis Hospital executive administrative assistants, Gloria Rojo, Laura Torres and Mary Bernal, for their generous help.

INTRODUCTION

James Madison, a founding father of our United States Constitution, once said:

> A popular government, without popular information, or the means of acquiring it, is but a prologue to a face or a tragedy; or, perhaps both. Knowledge will forever govern ignorance, and a people who mean to be their own Governors must arm themselves with the power which knowledge gives.

Over 200 years after liberating themselves from the yoke of governmental tyranny, the people of these United States of America must revolt again and wrench themselves from the bondage of medical ignorance. In his fantastic volume *Health in the 21st Century*, Francisco Contreras, MD, fights against conventional illiteracy to enlighten us against this country's newest tragedy. Our founding fathers have been turning over in their graves for too long. It's time now to arm ourselves, not with guns and bombs, but with the power of knowledge that Dr. Contreras, a brilliant writer, researcher and humanitarian, gives us in his landmark book.

Dr. Contreras uses the Don Quixote character in the book *Man From La Mancha* to characterize alternative medicine's battles against the conventional governmental agencies that protect pharmaceutical interests and corporate medical Goliath's.

They are giants and if you are afraid, don't get in my way,
and start praying in the meantime. I'm going to engage
them in fierce and unequal battle.
-Don Quixote, *Man From La Mancha*,
Miguel DeCervantes y Saavedra.

You'll be surprised by what you'll learn, fascinated by what you didn't know, and amazed that nobody is doing anything about it. Arm yourself so you may join a powerful, not-so-underground network of people determined to challenge the FDA—an authority that not only freely jeopardizes your health and the health of your loved ones, but acts unlawfully to stifle your freedom of speech, knowledge and medical choice.

Unencumbered by conventional ignorance and political correctness, the information contained in this incredible book will arm you with what you need to know so you can make responsible decisions about your and your family's health.

Read this book and LEARN about environmental enemies that threaten our health, the gross inadequacies of conventional medicine, how the food industry is ruled by money, not nutrition, the absolute necessity of nutritional supplementation, and the power of God to confront disease with great strength.

DISCOVER how nutrition can make our lives longer and better, which drugs and processed foods to avoid and why, why more and more doctors are prescribing alternative therapies, and who is profiting from dangerous medicine.

FIGHT DISEASE by discovering carefully hidden research elaborately buried and denied by convention but proven over and over through valid scientific testing and study by licensed, credential doctors and scientists. Dr. Contreras debunks commonly held beliefs about disease, and uncovers compelling evidence of governmental plots so insidious but plausible that they have to be true. After reading this book, you'll want to immediately contact your government representatives.

You'll want to DEMAND freedom of medical choice after reading how conventional medical "wisdom" promotes health- care dogma and effectively limits your viable and efficacious health-care choices. Health-care reform is a farce. We are being treated as subjects, not citizens. Only with a thorough, well-informed uprising of medical consumers will we win back the freedoms entrusted to us by our forefathers.

HELP YOURSELF with the positive information contained in this book, the benefits of nutritional supplementation and how it can help you reverse the chemical, informational and political poison forced on you and your loved ones daily.

I highly recommend this book, and I encourage all my friends, readers and followers to read it thoroughly. If you aren't already politically and medically active already, you will be after reading this book.

Maureen Kennedy Salaman

CONTENTS

Chapter 1

A Race Against Time

Chapter 2

Back to the Future

Chapter 3

Hunger Is Vicious

Chapter 4

111: The Doctor's Number

Chapter 5
The Possible Dream

Chapter 6
Neither Too Little Nor Too Much

Chapter 7
Between Heaven and Earth

Epilogue

References

Index

IN FRIENDSHIP

God gave each of us unique talents, gifts, and purposes. He sends many special people into our lives to help in our development. Without these special friends, none of us could be the person that God intended us to be. None of us could complete the mission that God entrusts to each of us. Though it is impossible for me to list all of the people who have played an important role in my life, I do want to mention:

Dr. Alexis and Virginia Setzer, Ricardo and Martalicia Zazueta, Senator Amador and Yamel Rodriguez, Agustin and Virginia Suarez, Brady and Cristina Fleck, Alex and Ana Phillips, Dr. J.F. Lagos, Dr. Antonio Jimenez, Dr. Ismael Cosio, Dr. Carlos Jimenez, Guadalupe Leon, Julio and Jenny Souza, Jorge Amezcua, Eduardo and Alejandra Ruiz, David and Laura Ruiz, Oliverio Ruiz, Ramon Rodriguez, Jose Flores, Francisco and Joyce Palau, Danny and Charise Vierra, Dr. Ramon Carrizales, Samuel and Ana Lia Bretts, Daniel Tochijara, Dr. Mary Ruth Swope, Dr. Mario Soto, Dr. Cal Streeter, Dr. Alex Duarte, Don and Carolyn Bird, Donald Factor, Charles Molina, Sarah Sackett, Thomas Frankito, James Bergstom, Mr. and Mrs. Eldon Jewett, Kathleen Jewett, Theresa Tamez, Beatriz Fimbres, Juan Alba, Dennis Itami, Ron Price, Ron Wright, Sharon Brooks, Rosa Garcia, Priscilla Breck, Paul Lehnert, Dr. Franco Eduardo Mendez, R. Russell and Norma Bixler, Evelynn Keen, Shary Oden, Lorraine Rosenthal, Peggy Pouson, Dr. Jonathan V. Wright, "Blackie" Gonzales, Dr. Trowbridge, Charlie Fox, Pam and Ellis Lowe, Dr. James Balch, Michael Sunstein, Lisa Elder, Erika Cervantes, Bob Martin, Julian Leon, and my brothers and sisters of San Pablo Evangelical Church.

IN GRATITUDE

There are those whom I particularly must thank for the powerful impact they had in my professional and personal life. Even 18 years since the departure to heaven of my eldest sister, Estela Contreras de Kennedy, her powerful love for the Lord and commitment to excellence in serving others still burns strong in my heart. I am grateful to Dr. Abel Mellado and his wife Rita, who is also my sister, and to Eliud Elizondo and his wife Eva, another of my sisters. These two families worked with my father from the beginning, and stood firmly by him through the years of persecution. Pastor Joel Ordaz and his wife Ana, still another sister, took the evangelistic ministry at Oasis to a higher level. Rev. David and Linda Kennedy have always been a spiritual rock to all our family. Today, all four families are committed full time to the ministry, and lead important Christian congregations in Mexico and the United States. My brother, Dr. Ernesto Contreras, Jr., is an inspiration for his wealth of knowledge and his dedication to the healing mission. With the loving support of his wife Lety, he spends much of his time writing Christian books and preaching the Gospel.

I cannot thank all my patients enough for the impact they have had on my life. It is because of them that I continue to search for an answer to illness and ways to prevent others from falling into the grip of disease and other adversaries of health.

Most of all, I want to thank my wife Rosy for her undivided support, encouragement, input and love. I thank my daughters, Rosa Estela, Marcela, Sandra and Debora for the incredible blessing and inspiration they are to me. Thank You, God, for all, especially for the gift of salvation through Jesus Christ.

PLEASE NOTE

The information presented in this book is not intended to prevent, inhibit or detain anyone from seeking out and/or receiving proper medical diagnosis and treatment for any health condition, nor is it intended to replace or supplant any medical treatment. Everyone should seek two or more professional opinions before any medical treatment or lifestyle changes are undertaken.

This book is strictly for the reader's information. Any and all therapies, doctors or facilities should be researched before making an informed and personal decision as to what medical treatments to initiate. This book sets forth the opinion of only the author.

FOREWORD

"The times, they are a changin'…" These lyrics written by Bob Dylan in the early 60s have never been more relevant. Something very significant is happening in the world of health care today. Almost daily we read newspaper articles relating some new study showing the benefits of vitamins, minerals, antioxidants or other "phytochemicals" in our search for longevity and a better quality of life. Alongside these nutritional discoveries, we read about such sophisticated developments as genetic engineering, laser surgery and yet another round of pharmaceuticals promising nearly miraculous cures for everything from obesity to cancer. Without question, the next 20 years will bring amazing and profound discoveries that will impact health care as we know it.

Yet, some claim that these new discoveries are not new at all. They point to years of research by unorthodox researchers who herald a need to move away from our dependence on drugs, radiation and excessive surgeries. They cite substantial success in treating degenerative diseases with nutritional, detoxification and other therapies. They point out that the Establishment is at least 20 years behind in understanding and promoting the benefits of lifestyle changes.

As health care consumers, most of us fall between these two camps of contesting philosophies. We desperately want to trust our doctors, hospitals and governmental agencies in matters related to health. Yet, we are shocked to find that the medical profession's own publications, such as the *Journal of the American Medical Association* and the *New England Journal of Medicine*, unapologetically report that over 100,00 Americans die each year because of something a doctor did to them while in the hospital, that close to 50 percent of all deaths on the operating table are caused by the very folks who are supposed to be saving our lives, and that the vast majority of oncologists would not personally accept the treatments they continue to prescribe for their patients. What has gone wrong with health care today?

As we move toward the 21st Century, who can help us sort through the opposing arguments that are gathering momentum? Who can combine a respect for the work of alternative healers with the sophistication of modern science and help chart a course for our future? I believe that Francisco Contreras, MD, from the Oasis of Hope Hospital, can. Dr. Contreras was educated as a medical doctor in the United States and Mexico, and specialized in surgery at the world famous University Hospital in Vienna, Austria. Dr. Contreras brings a unique blend of wisdom and insight to the debate currently raging over health and health care for the future.

There are three reasons why I believe that Dr. Francisco Contreras is uniquely qualified to speak with authority on issues that will touch every one of our lives. First, Francisco is a faithful protégé of his father, Ernesto Contreras, Sr., MD, who has served as a pathologist and oncologist for more than fifty years. While many others enter the medical profession for financial reward, Ernesto Contreras, Sr., has served selflessly, many times setting aside his reputation and personal gain because of his deeply held belief that "a doctor should love his patient as he loves himself." Ernesto Contreras, Sr. is one of the great pioneering heroes for health care in the 20th century, but who has gone largely unnoticed because he places the patient above politics and economics. My visits to the Oasis of Hope Hospital have convinced me that Francisco is following closely in his father's footsteps. His commitment to excellence in his areas of specialty, and his obvious compassion for his patients are tributes to the example his father has set.

Second, Francisco is an articulate and well-educated spokesperson for what is happening now and for what should happen in the future to make health care better. He is a great communicator, capable of translating complex scientific information into language easy for the lay person to understand and, even better, to apply immediately for a better quality of life. Francisco's engaging personality has made him a popular speaker at a wide variety of events across North America over the last decade.

Last, and most important in my thinking, Francisco Contreras is particularly qualified to be a bridge between scientific medicine and alternative medicine because he is a servant. His love for God, family and patients is quickly recognized and consistent in each of the many hats he wears. I would not hesitate to put myself under his care, and that is more than I can say about many so-called experts. Francisco is a person uniquely prepared for such a time as this. His insights and recommendations in *Health In the 21st Century* are right on target. All who follow his advice will take a significant step toward what we all wish for... a long and healthy life.

Health In the 21st Century is filled with valuable information and recommendations on how you can enjoy better health. If you are facing a health crisis, this book will help you navigate the many treatment options that are yours (even when your doctor claims there is only one). If you are healthy, this book provides very important information that will help you keep your health and keep it for a long time! For those who have ears to hear, *Health In The 21st Century* has some very significant things to say. It holds the potential to change your life forever!

Ron Price

Chapter 1

A Race Against Time

Men talk of killing time, while time quietly kills them.

Dion Boucicault

The Link Between Life and Death

Occasionally it's abrupt and merciful, sometimes covert and agonizing, and in rare instances, in the midst of pain, even welcome —Death, the ultimate triumph of disease, is a reality that all want to avoid or at least postpone. To talk about health without considering disease is like speaking about air and forgetting to mention oxygen. They are inseparable ideas because they are pitted against each other. Regardless of our religious or cultural backgrounds, we all share the love of life and the desire to prolong it as long as possible.

The medical industry's propaganda has impregnated our minds with the idea that highly qualified doctors aided by monstrous scientific and technological advances have subdued disease: our world is safe, thanks to them. Unquestionably impressive achievements have been made in the modern medical indus-try, but they are sadly darkened by the ample and frightful fail-ures.

The fight against disease is based on a nearsighted vision that, as we will see, has taken many lives. We have fought with commitment and valor, but against the wrong enemy unfortu-nately. Omission is our sin. We have overlooked obvious, simple things that profoundly affect the health of all.

There is no question that the length of one's life is directly connected to one's physical health. The simplest definition of health, according to most physicians, is the absence of dis-ease. However, this seems shallow if we compare it with the 2500-year-old definition of Hippocrates, the father of medi-cine: "Health is the perfect balance between man and his en-vironment." If such a balance could exist, would immortality be possible?

Immortality

From the Biblical point of view, Adam and Eve enjoyed the cleanest, most unpolluted environment ever in Eden. This perfect balance with their environment was not threatened by disease or death. In Eden, however, there was one stipulation: that they refrain from eating the fruit from a single tree. "But of the tree of the knowledge of good and evil, you shall not eat. For in the day that you eat of it, you will surely die." (Genesis 2:17)

However, neither Adam nor Eve fell instantly dead after eating that apple. What happened? In my opinion, in the instant they ate of the forbidden fruit, they had sinned, and the perfect balance was lost. The path to death was then opened in both the physical and spiritual worlds.

According to the Bible the cycle of life experienced a dramatic paradigm shift. Before, we were born to live forever, but now we are born, we grow, we reproduce ourselves, and we die. This life cycle is deeply rooted in our minds after centuries of experience. So why do we still search for the fountain of youth? Because very deeply ingrained in our genes is the information that we were created to be immortal.

The Mercedes-Benz company, in an advertisement, shows one of its motor cars built in 1955 which, after all these years, shows an odometer reading of 1,000,000 miles.

Its owner still enjoys the benefits of his investment. Now I don't doubt that the Germans produce excellent motor cars. However, if the car in the advertisement were a Ford built in Mexico, and if it received the necessary maintenance and replacement parts, this modest little car would also run indefinitely.

The marvelous thing about our body is that it has the power to furnish its own spare parts. The body's ability to replace expired cells is the miracle of life and is the trace of immortality that was not lost in Eden. If our body did not have the capacity to regenerate its tissues, we would not live very long. For example, if our body failed to replace red blood cells, we would die in about four months.

Within the extremely complicated organization of our body, each cell has a different cycle that lasts from hours to years. Some neurons may accompany us for most of our lives, but the remainder of our cells are constantly being replaced. For example, the liver we had a few months ago is not the one we have now, because all the cells within it are new. The same thing is true of all the organs. If this regeneration was uninterrupted—if it were not impeded— we would be immortal. Immortality was definitively lost at some point after the creation, but certain traces of it still remain. Historical records indicate that we can at least enjoy spectacular longevity. Some Biblical characters like Moses, the liberator of the Jewish people, lived 120 years. Even as death approached him, the Biblical record states that his eyes were not dim nor had he lost his vigor (Deuteronomy 44:7). Abraham lived 175 years (Genesis 25:8). Even more surprising is the case of his wife Sarah who, though living only 127 years (Genesis 23:1), gave birth at 91 years of age (Genesis 21:1-8). The man who lived longest on the face of the earth was Methuselah, Noah's grandfather. He lived for 969 years (Genesis 5:21).

In an era like ours, time is a valuable commodity. Due in part to the great number of activities we would like to engage in, and to the fact that time often gets away from us, living 969 years would be more than a luxury. Think how many careers we could pursue, how many times we could travel around the world, and how much we could learn!

Some foolish critics consider many of the stories in the Sacred Book to be within the realm of myth. However, it is worth the trouble to ask ourselves whether the environmental conditions in the past might have made it possible to live a long time.

The ecosystem before the flood, according to many experts, was extraordinarily human friendly, but we have lost that perfect balance with our world. At the present moment, such an environment is difficult for even the mentally gifted to imagine.

Apparently, we have no choice but to grit our teeth and face up to death, but many prefer to fight it. This resolve to battle death was beautifully expressed by the poet Dylan Thomas when he said, "Do not go gently into that goodnight. Rage, rage against the dying of the light." The human being doesn't allow itself to be defeated. As this century ends, scientists dream of ways to prolong life.

Time Waits For No Man

> Clock! Cease mocking the hours because my
> life is ending.
> **Roberto Cantoral**

"Life is very, very short," says Dr. Souresh Rattan of Aarhus University Denmark. "At age 50, just when we have learned how to live, just when we are ready to give something back to society, we begin to fall apart. What a loss!"

More than one of us will agree with Dr. Rattan, even though we may not have reached 50. In 1513, Ponce De Leon accompanied Hernan Cortez on his second expedition to America, because he had heard that the fountain of youth could be found in Florida. He lost his life in the search for this marvel. If he could return to life, this visionary explorer would be flabbergasted to find the extraordinary tools present-day scientists use in the exploration of immortality.

Research for a means to live longer has never been abandoned. There are the legitimate efforts of modern scientists on the one hand and the ridiculous practices of fanatics on the other. For example, there are people who have had themselves cryogenically frozen in the hopes that the future will yield a cure for the disease from which they suffer. Making use of scientific methods much more ingenious and sophisticated, modern day Ponce De Leons study the why of aging and explore the possibility of reversing the aging process. At the moment, the most important and surprising findings have been in the area of nutrition (surprising?).

If we nourish ourselves adequately, we could prolong our lives 30 to 35 years, and if the genetic mechanisms that control aging can be discovered, life could be extended for one hundred, two hundred, or five hundred years. Dr. William Regelson of the Medical College of Virginia says that in light of recent discoveries we should be able to add thirty healthy years to human life within the next decade. Furthermore, as we learn to control the genes involved in aging, the possibilities for prolonging life seem practically limitless. A philosophical and good friend of mine, Ricardo Zazueta, heard me speak of these probable accomplishments, and commented in a perturbed way, "How awful! Imagine the boredom! The horror of living with the same mother-in-law all those years."

We don't know to what extent scientists will be able to reverse the mechanisms of aging and prolong life. The fact of the matter is that investigations of this biological puzzle are ongoing in hundreds of universities in the United States, Europe, and Asia. In California, for example, one scientist has discovered the genes that cause the aging of skin. In Texas, a group of researchers discovered a way to make hundreds of cells reproduce themselves indefinitely. Several groups have discovered genes that prolong life and those that shorten it. Others have detected the switches that turn genes on and off. Biologists have been able to double and triple the life of insects and the life of red blood cells in human beings.

Of course, in the scientific fields there are those who oppose the project to prolong human life, or who voice great skepticism. These critics imagine all the disastrous consequences that would accompany the prolonging of life. Excess worldwide population, economic insolvency, and a devastated environment are a few of the problems they foresee.

I look at the possibility of prolonged life more optimistically, since we would surely find better solutions to the world's problems offered by people with the wisdom and the maturity that longer life provides. Even with all the possible complications, the idea of living a lot longer than we now live is difficult to cast aside.

In the Roman Empire, the average life span was twenty-two years. In 1850, people from the United States died at around forty-five years of age. At present, the average life span in the United States is seventy-five years. Today in this country there are 46,000 persons who are 100 years or older. It is predicted that by the year 2020 this number will increase to 266,000.

There is no doubt that longevity has improved impressively, but there is not necessarily a corresponding quality of life. The death of the elderly is usually preceded by at least twenty years of illness. The true secret of prolonging life would be found in the regulating of the genes that determine longevity and those that control the breakdown of the body.

In 1962, the Nobel Prize for Medicine was awarded to John Watson, Francis Crick, and Maurice Wilkins for having discovered the structure of DNA, the substance found in cells which contains hereditary information. From that point, biologists and other scientists began to ask themselves if the body contained a biological clock that determines when the human being should begin to age. Doctors Calvin Harley Carol Greider and Bruce Futcher found a genetic mechanism that functions as a clock.

The ticking of this clock depends on the length of the telomers, long threads which carry an important genetic message which causes cells to regenerate.

When a cell divides, it loses from five to twenty segments of the telomers. When all the segments are depleted, the message is interrupted and the cell ceases to regenerate itself. Therefore, the length of these threads determines how long a cell family will live.

Furthermore, the loss of the telomers in cellular division may contribute to the development of diseases such as arteriosclerosis osteoarthritis, osteoporosis, and diabetes mellitus. Scientists believe that if it were possible to control the disintegration of the telomers so as to retard aging, a higher quality of life would be realized because such diseases would be slowed considerably. Could the telomers be the punishment that Adam and Eve received?

Scientists know that there is a close relationship between the chromosomes and the genes, which are the building blocks of DNA. In order to understand this relationship, it is helpful to imagine a ladder. Each gene would represent a rung, and the chromosomes would be the rails. All species have their hereditary information coded in the genes.

Understand that God created the chromosomes to function as a computer program whose start-up instructions are written in the genes. When the chromosomes get instructions from the genes, the program begins to run. Amino acids come together and form proteins, which in turn combine to form cells, which come together to form a plant, animal, or human being, according to the blueprint found in the chromosome's program. The same chromosomes and genes are going to determine the peculiarities of each of their products depending on the information they may carry. Thus, in human beings they will determine stature, eye color, IQ, temperament, vocational tendencies, and so on. We can affirm that all the information about our lives is written in the DNA.

We possess a total of forty-six types of chromosomes. A surprising discovery with respect to chromosomes was that of Dr. Carl Barrett, who discovered that chromosome 1 promotes aging. Dr. James Smith and Dr. Olivia Smith found that chromosome 4 does the same. Dr. Michael West discovered genes that initiate the aging process in skin cells, blood vessels, and the brain.

At the University of Texas Southwestern Medical Center, Dr. W. Wright and Dr. Shay discovered two genetic programs, which they called mortality one and mortality two. Upon activating mortality one, the cell gradually begins to age. When mortality two goes into action, the cell degenerates rapidly and soon dies. Upon deactivating mortality one, scientists could extend the life of a cell in culture between 40 percent and 100 percent. Nevertheless, sooner or later mortality two was activated and the cells began to decay. When the scientists detained mortality two, the cells began to reproduce indefinitely — they became immortal.

Now the task is to discover if this reproduction can be controlled. Our bodies are predetermined by genetic information, and each person develops in conformity with the blueprints in his genes. In this process, there is a sophisticated balance between the powerful stage of growth and the regulatory stage. If these opposing forces didn't exist in the universe, or in human beings, nature would be a monstrous disaster. Imagine what life would be like if we didn't have the genes that regulated the size of our nose, feet, or height. We would be truly horrible looking creatures.

Genetic research has brought us amazing discoveries like mortality one and mortality two. Unfortunately, the benefits of these discoveries seem out of reach to us. However, the same experimentation has brought excellent practical applications that are now within our grasp.

Thanks to genetic engineering, hormones like insulin, which once before were difficult to produce, can now be made very easily. Scientists can "teach" bacteria how to manufacture these products. Scientists transfer the pertinent genetic information to the bacteria, and the bacteria begin to cost-effectively produce the hormone. Antibiotics, enzymes and other medicines are being produced in much the same way. Other bacteria are trained to eat petroleum to clean up oil spills like that of the Exxon Valdez.

Yet, all these advances have their risks and costs, to say nothing of the danger of toying with the creation process. What happens when we decide to play God? The fact is, the majority of this genetic research is performed in a laboratory. Scientists know that what happens there doesn't necessarily occur in real life. In my opinion, we are far from the practical applications of this genetic information and, therefore, far from slowing the aging process.

The Third Age

Still, researchers press on in their efforts to prolong life and control disease. The presence or absence of disease determines the quality of life in the third age, which begins for most of us at sixty. In this third age, we lose approximately 40 percent of the functional capacities we possessed when we were between 25 and 30 years of age.

The deterioration is primarily physical. For example, there is a decalcification of the bones and a diminishing of the cartilage, in conjunction with a reduction in stature. This, coupled with muscular flaccidity, creates problems in motor coordination, agility and equilibrium. When we experience these changes, it is not uncommon for us to fall down more often and to suffer injury from those falls.

Another example is the fact that the lungs transport less oxygen to the cells as we get older. The lack of oxygen, among other things, slows the burning of glucose. This operation is fundamental to the body's production of energy. Therefore, we tend to have less energy as we age.

In addition, there is a greater accumulation of fat in the whole organism, especially the arteries in the form of arteriosclerosis. The consequences of this hardening of the arteries are bad circulation and slower transportation of nutrients to the cells. The heart pumps less blood to the brain, producing cerebral dysfunction, impaired mental agility, loss of memory and senility.

These physiological changes provoke the psychological consequences of anxiety and depression. Good heavens! Much of this sounds like symptoms many of us are already experiencing, and we are not yet forty-five. The following are some of the various theories of the aging process.

As It Is Written

Humans, like other creatures of the animal kingdom, have been designed to reproduce their kind and see their progeny become independent. The fact that some people may live longer than the rest of us only confirms that human development, from cradle to grave, is determined by a genetic clock that signals the various stages of the aging process. Aging is a genetically programmed process, just as infancy or adolescence.

Neural Extinction

At birth, a person possesses some twelve billion neurons. Unlike other types of cells, neurons do not reproduce themselves or, if they do, the process is very slow. In the course of our lives we lose a large percentage of neurons. Some researchers theorize that the main cause of aging could be this neuron loss, because the brain controls all organs and their functions. The neuron loss causes the brain to produce a hormone which decreases the body's ability to consume oxygen. This interferes with the synthesis of proteins and cell division. Nevertheless, opponents of this theory point out that even species lacking a neuron system as complex as ours age in a way very similar to the way humans age.

Rust Never Sleeps: Free Radicals

Other scientists have a different perspective of the aging process. According to Dr. Denham Harman, emeritus professor of the University of Nebraska, aging arises from the process of oxidization. We have all observed how a peeled apple turns brown, or how an abandoned car corrodes over time. These are the result of oxidization. We use the term rust to refer to oxidization of metals.

The aging process is similar to what happens to apples and metal in the presence of oxygen. Certainly, cells must have a source of energy in order to maintain life, and that source is oxygen. But oxygen is a double-edged sword. It maintains life, but at the same time it can be very destructive. If a person breathed pure oxygen for two days, instead of air which contains only 21 percent oxygen, he would die because his lungs would be destroyed.

By 1954, Dr. Harman's research had led him to postulate his theory of aging – that free radicals, the byproducts of oxidation, are the true cause of aging. This theory is now widely accepted in the United States and, indeed, the whole world.

What Are Free Radicals?

Free radicals are among the agents most capable of damaging an organism on the biochemical plane. Free radicals are formed within the organism itself as a result of the conversion of sugar and oxygen into energy. Conversion takes place in the mitochondria, structures found inside cells. Mitochondria fulfill their function of producing energy, but leave free radicals in their wake.

Like many other substances, free radicals carry out a beneficial function in the organism. They assist in the extermination of germs and certain bacteria, but they can also cause serious damage to the body. When free radicals accumulate, they cause chain reactions that damage cell membranes and genetic material.

In nature, electrons exist as pairs in the orbits of nuclei. These electron pairs lose a partner in the oxidization process. An atom or nucleus that has lost an electron partner is called a free radical.

Energy is produced when an oxygen molecule loses an electron. The process destabilizes the molecule, like a balloon that deflates when its knot is untied. In its wild flight, the freed electron (free radical) seeks to unite with another electron to stabilize itself. The liberated electron resolves its problem by stealing an electron from another molecule.

This causes a chain reaction resulting in cellular chaos. The molecules strike furiously against each other in an effort to stabilize themselves, further destabilizing other molecules within the cell. Once the process begins, it is difficult to control. It is hard to imagine that such devastation begins in these tiny little molecules that live only a few thousandths of a second. Yet every chromosome in our body receives some ten thousand attacks daily.

Free radicals also interrupt other cellular and enzymatic processes such as hormonal regulation and the development of the proteins necessary to regulate nerves, muscles, skin, and hair. The destructive capacity of the free radicals is enormous, especially because they alter genetic codes. A single free radical can damage a million or more molecules.

Free radicals cause a multitude of diseases, including arteriosclerosis, Alzheimer's disease, cancer, high blood pressure, schizophrenia, Parkinson's disease, Down's syndrome, memory loss, brain deficiencies, paralysis, cataracts, arthritis, emphysema, and cystic fibrosis. Without a doubt, free radicals sabotage good health, and encourage aging. I will explain in chapter six what we can do to combat free radicals.

Every Good Thing Comes To an End

Our bodies regenerate by cell division, the mechanism by which our cells reproduce themselves. As we advance in years, our cells don't reproduce themselves as easily as they did when we were younger. In addition, with each cell division, the risk of error in the reproductive process increases. The inevitable errors result in degeneration and the development of diseases that undermine our health.

For example, cells can become cancerous if their genetic mechanism fails to follow its precise instructions. When our body reconstructs areas where there are large quantities of dead and defective cells, the oncogenes activate neoplastic cells, which have a very rapid reproductive rate. To avoid the formation of tumors, these cells are regulated by tumor suppressing genes, which ensure that tissue will grow to exactly the required degree.

This mechanism is effectively and unceasingly carried out from birth. Sadly, with the passage of years, this genetic process is exposed to the damaging effects of free radicals and other contaminants. When the process fails to operate exactly as it should, degeneration and diseases undermine health, and the door to aging is opened wide.

The Enemy Within

With the passage of time, our organism finds it increasingly difficult to eliminate waste materials produced within the body, environmental waste and contaminants. For example, as cells synthesize complex substances from simpler ones —a process called metabolism— they produce toxins that oxidize the proteins. The cells and their organs deteriorate because these waste products and toxins aren't eliminated. We go through life accumulating the toxins which eventually stifle vital functions and cause degeneration.

Inadequate Protection

We possess 70 million different antibodies which protect us from internal and external invaders. This incredible immune system is regulated by means of electromagnetic and chemical processes designed to recognize enemies. With time, this once powerful defense system becomes vulnerable to the viruses, toxins and contaminants that attack our bodies.

On occasion, these attacks are so aggressive and frequent that the defense mechanisms are overwhelmed. If the chemical, biological, and emotional stresses are too great, the organism's immune system will become so disoriented that it will attack its own cells resulting in auto-immune disorders such as arthritis, lupus and diabetes. Although old age predisposes us to these complications, they can occur in earlier stages of life.

The Sweet Life

An excess of sugar in the body, especially refined sugar, causes proteins within the cells to stick to each other, a phenomenon called cross-bonding. With time, this cross-bonding causes hardening of the joints, loss of flexibility of the blood vessels, and fragile bones. Cross-bonding ultimately causes diseases such as diabetes, arteriosclerosis, kidney disease and pulmonary disease.

Use It or Lose It

The excessive use or disuse of the body also plays a role in the aging process. Two hundred years ago, exercise was unavoidable because most people survived by the sweat of their brow. Today, exercise is viewed by enthusiasts as a recreational activity, and by the general public as a form of torture. Let's face it: Technological advances are focused on saving us time and effort.

The body experiences maximum physical capacity when it is between 25 and 30 years old. From then, it travels a regressive journey, one that is accelerated if we avoid physical activity. Aerobics, jogging, walking and sports activity slow down the process of deterioration by some 20 percent. Nevertheless, excessive physical activity can also shorten one's life. For example, professional football players have life expectancies shorter than that of the average person.

What You Eat Can Kill You

Can a person's diet accelerate aging? The answer is yes. All bodily functions depend on a steady supply of the elements needed to sustain those functions. Although some of the elements are produced internally, most of them are obtained from the food we eat.

In spite of the body's incredible capabilities, it is often impossible for it to convert junk [food] and chemicals into fuel that will power bodily functions. On the contrary, these poisons promote deterioration and an acceleration of the aging process. We can't stop aging by eating better foods, but we can certainly slow it down.

Each of the proponents of the theories of aging give an explanation regarding the shortness of life. Although a combination of these theories gives a global vision of mortality and immortality, the genetic code seems to have the most power over the aging process.

The Exception To The Rule

I was once invited to a show at which the famous comedian George Burns was to be interviewed. Mr. Burns was ninety years old. The dialogue between the interviewer and Mr. Burns, plus or minus a few words ran as follows,

Q: George, tell us, do you smoke a lot?

GB: Do I smoke? The only time I'm not smoking is when I'm asleep.

Q: Is it true that you also have a drinking habit?

GB: Well, you tell me. I drink about a liter of liquor a day.

Q: Do you engage in any type of exercise?

GB: Never.

Q: Well, what does your doctor say about that?

GB: I don't know what he would say. He's already dead.

The spectators, of course, saw the irony in Burns' words and almost burst their sides laughing. It is evident that, with time, the human body loses the ability to repair and defend itself. Consequently, it slowly declines. The wear and tear varies from person to person, according to their genetic structure. Burns was an exception to the rule. He was gifted with super-genes and an immunilogical army of Rambos capable of resisting twelve hours of cigar smoke and a liter of liquor a day.

At the other extreme, who among of us has not heard about some health nut, obsessively preoccupied with nutrition and exercise, who died young of cancer or a heart attack? Burns and the health fanatic represent the exceptions, of course. Most of us are somewhere in between these two extremes.

You've No One But Yourself To Blame

We should accept the responsibility for the care of our own health. Most of us desire a gratifyingly long, ailment-free life. There is no way to achieve this other than to do things that are good for our health and to avoid practices that cause our bodies to deteriorate. Proponents of theories believe them to be completely true. Yet, they remain theories —neither proven nor disproven. I will summarize them in two parts:

I.   Undeniably, our organism is controlled by growth and growth-inhibiting factors. When we are young, our body obviously has an abundance of growth factors which permit the body to grow rapidly. At physical maturity, we possess the same number of growth factors and growth-inhibiting factors. As the years pass, the balance changes. The growth factors diminish and the growth-inhibitors increase. Lost cells are replaced by fewer fresh cells and the aging process begins.

II.   Our organism requires certain resources for the reconstruction of cells. The codes for cellular reconstruction can be in perfect order, but the quality of the cell generated depend on the quality of its constituent amino acids, vitamins, minerals and so forth. These nutrients require the energy from carbohydrates, proteins and fats. If these elements are lacking, or if there is insufficient energy to power them, the reconstruction process is less than adequate. In this way, too, the aging process is accelerated.

The body's biochemical processes are not unlike the building of a house. Imagine that you just finished building the house of your dreams. Then for some reason you are forced to move to a far away place like central Africa. However, you have the blueprints and a list of all the materials, so you merrily resolve to build it again in Africa.

Upon arriving in central Africa you will experience a major setback. No Home Depot! Not all the materials you need are available and those you can find are not of the same quality as those manufactured in your country. This doesn't mean you can't build a house. However, it does mean that your replacement house, in spite of the fact that the same blueprint was used, will not compare to the original because of the limited supplies and the inferior quality of the materials used.

The same is true of our bodies. Although all our chromosomes and genes bear all the correct codes and information necessary for the building of replacement cells, if the elements provided to the organism are of inferior quality, the organism will produce replacement cells of increasingly inferior quality. Physical degeneration is the consequence of eating foods of inferior quality that have been stripped of their necessary nutrients.

In the same way that a house is only as good as the quality of its materials, the body is only as strong as the quality of the nutrients it receives. If a house has a strong foundation, it can resist external disturbances. However, if the quality of the foundation is poor, or if the foundation is poorly laid, the house may fall. So it is that a deficiency of one nutrient can cause illness, and the absence of a single nutrient can cause death.

In my opinion then, the best strategy for slowing the aging process is nutrition. Even after so much technological effort in the search for the fountain of youth, experts now tell us that we can better the quality of life and prolong our existence by fixing our eyes on nature. They tell us we can slow the aging process by nourishing ourselves with organic fruits, vegetables, and grains that have not been manipulated by man. That is to say, our food must be eaten as God put it in the world, without alteration. My grandmother knew that —she lived almost 90 excellent years, and she didn't spend billions of your tax dollars on "life saving" research.

Theories of aging oblige us to remember that we were designed to live longer than we do. Life is too short to fulfill all our dreams. I support research that seeks ways to prolong life. I don't necessarily hope that we can live one hundred, three hundred, or five hundred years, but I do hope that we can live through our third age with a lucid, joyous and buoyant spirit, and enjoy good physical health. The elderly population of the United States is growing fast, but it cannot take care of itself. Adequate nutrition, exercise and avoidance of junk food are easy and cost effective measures we can do to improve and prolong our health.

With a few exceptions, prolonged health is a personal responsibility. It is something we strive for, not something that is given to us. But good health pertains not only to our body, it encompasses the emotional and spiritual spheres, aspects that are often ignored by physicians. Although many scientists and patients, and most of society, are looking for and even demanding change, doctors continue to resist it. The complex task of building solid health has many enemies. Defeating these enemies begins with knowing who and what they are. I do not want doctors to be considered an enemy but I'm afraid that if doctors are not willing to break paradigms and adopt a wellness approach, we will have to put them on the endangered species' list.

Chapter 2

Back to the Future

Our World

> The beauty of the world . . . has two edges, one of laughter, one of
> anguish, cutting the heart asunder.
>
> **Virginia Woolf**

We are all aware of the differences that exist between man
and animals, the principle one being that God has endowed us
with a spirit. Among other things, this spirit is what gives
us the capacity to consciously alter the environment
to meet our needs. Animals and plants, on the other

hand, adapt to the environment instinctively and submissively.

It is necessary that humans manipulate the environment. After all, we do not adapt to extreme weather conditions as well as other species do. For example, we don't have a heavy, thermal hide like bears. Therefore, if we don't cut down a tree and build a fire in the snowy mountains, we will freeze to death.

Unfortunately, we not only make the changes required in order to subsist, we also criminally strip the rest of the ecosystem to improve our level of comfort. From the beginning of this millennium, we have been conscious of this damage and we know it will come back to haunt us. Nevertheless, just as drug addicts will consciously choose to destroy their bodies to satisfy the craving, so we destroy the ecosystem to satisfy our desire for pleasure and comfort.

Humanity demands the comfort and convenience that accompany modernization even when aware of the high price to be paid by generations to come. We are daily reminded in the news of the problems related to contamination and environmental destruction, but in the face of all this, we are passive and most of us do nothing about it. I must confess that I personally feel uneasy when I encounter reports of this destruction in the newspaper or elsewhere.

In the first place, such information is hard to stomach because enough tragedy already takes place around me in the lives of my patients, many of whom are sentenced to die hopelessly from cancer. My time and effort are taken up in trying to defeat this disease and give hope to people who have lost heart. In the second place, it irritates me when information is distorted to serve the agenda of some special interest group.

Yet, the media does allow us glimpses of a reality that is around us. We have a responsibility to take off our blinders, yet it doesn't do any good to recognize what is happening all around the world if we don't lift a finger to solve the problems in our own neighborhoods. I'm not suggesting that we lose all feeling for those suffering famine in Somalia or India. However, I am asserting that we show genuine concern for our own children, who are living in an environment so disastrous that it presents a real threat to the quality of their lives today.

The Past In The present

In 1982, I was invited to an Amish community to give a lecture on alternative therapies against cancer. The further I moved into this community, the more I felt I was traveling in a time machine. Who doesn't remember the adventures of H.G. Wells and his fabulous machine? I traveled into what seemed like 17th century America. There were fewer paved roads and I began to see only horse-drawn carriages.

The people's black attire reminded me of movies about the first immigrants from England. These pleasant people not only introduced me to their community, they also demonstrated the true meaning of love and respect for nature. It is my impression, that the Amish are an ultraconservative Christian religion that tries to live life by Biblical principles. In fact, all their communal laws have been based on the Sacred Text. I was surprised to discover that their garments were very modest and similar in style, like a uniform.

The Amish do everything by hand and by the sweat of the brow. They eat mainly what the earth produces without changing it any more than absolutely necessary for their sustenance. They do not have their water piped into the community, nor do they have sewer drains, gas, nor any kind of diesel or gasoline powered machines or electricity. They really do work from sun to sun.

After my lecture, I conversed a bit with them, asking why they chose this complicated and primitive lifestyle, especially since the advances of the 20th century have made life so much easier. As diplomatically as possible, I commented that it seemed a waste to reject the technological advances achieved by the intelligence that God has given man. They answered that they were convinced that in technological progress and industrial advance was the downfall of man physically, morally and spiritually. The profundity of this simple concept really impressed me, and my respect for their discipline, sacrifice and dedication to Biblical principle was deepened.

The truth doesn't hurt, but it does makes us uncomfortable. What argument could I propose? In everyone's consciousness without a doubt is the conviction that the industrial and technological revolution is killing us.

It is no accident that the Amish enjoy a life span some eight years longer than the average American. The night I spent in their community seemed to last an eternity. I was amazed at how difficult it was to be stripped of modern technology. I could not turn on a light to read, listen to a stereo, answer a telephone, or watch television the entire time I was there. It was a rare experience living with the Amish for 36 hours. I couldn't stop mulling over the lessons I had learned. Yet, I couldn't wait to check into a hotel, take a hot bath and not have to haul water from a well to wash my hands or flush the toilet.

As I write this on my multi-media, internet capable computer with CD Rom, Fax/Modem port, sound system, active matrix screen, and ink jet color printer, I am overcome by a terrible sense of guilt. Would I be willing to leave this and other comforts to help save our world? On one hand, the terrible present condition of the environment overwhelms me (contaminated rivers and lakes, a gigantic hole in the ozone layer, garbage everywhere, toxic waste that undermine health). Yet, I admire the incredible way that those technological advances increase productivity and contribute to the development of individuals and communities, and in some ways, elevate the quality and usefulness of our existence.

The ideal thing would be to maintain a balance between the benefits and the price of technology. Up to now, man has not been able to obtain balance on this plane. Out of reverence for comfort, we have permitted progress to continue on a destructive path. A reflection on the present situation of our environment should inspire us to do something to restore it. Let's not forget the urgent words of John F. Kennedy pronounced in a speech in 1963, "the supreme reality of our time is the vulnerability of our planet."

The Environment and Governmental Protection Agencies

Lift up your eyes to the heavens and look below to the earth for the heavens shall be undone like smoke and the world shall become like a garment and in the same way shall those that dwell therein perish.

Isaiah 51:6

God used the prophet Isaiah to give us both sublime messages and at the same time strong admonitions. His prophecy about the destruction of the planet while too advanced for his time was terribly accurate. It shows us that we should have been concerned for our environment for the last two millennia.

Unfortunately, ancient leaders, like modern ones, never imposed preventative measures. Rather, they waited for disaster to occur, then established methods for fixing the damage done.

Yet, there are examples of good efforts. When Paris was founded more than 2000 years ago, wastes were biodegradable and sewage filtered naturally into the groundwater. This water returned to the Seine River in a fairly clean state. Until the Middle Ages, the city continued to pour its residual waters into fields or into the streets. As the population increased, this practice became a severe public health problem. So, in 1200, the streets of Paris were paved and in the middle of each street, channels were built to drain away the sewage. In 1273, London imposed laws to protect the inhabitants from contamination. History shows that severe penalties were applied to those who did not obey such laws. For example, in 1306 a person was executed for burning coal in a restricted area.

In 1700, the Italian Bernardino Ramacini, after 40 years of research, reported in his work, *Diatribe of Occupational Diseases*, that a strict relationship existed between diseases and work conditions. The idea of conducting this research came to him while he observed the deplorable physical condition of workers who cleaned the sewers. He classified diseases according to the nature of the trade or profession and the elements to which they were exposed. He included all kinds of occupations (including sedentary ones such as clerks and writers and even the office of the Prince). His impressive research demonstrated the need for the government to form standards for work environments.

In the 18th century, Europeans, having battled the spread of the bubonic plague with a massive quarantine, were disposed to take necessary measures to ensure the public's health. The German Johan Peterfranc began to publish a work entitled *System For A Complete Medical Policy* in 1779, a treatise that took in all the aspects of social medicine. It was based on the research of illustrious men, from various European countries, regarding the principles and measures that prevailed in manners of public health.

Motivated by the cholera plague in 1851, the first international sanitation conference was convened in Paris. The most valuable fruit of this conference was the formulation of an international code for the prevention of pestilence, like cholera and yellow fever. It was in this part of the 19th century that hygiene was defined.

Another event which contributed to the health of the general public in the 19th century was the introduction of methods for the purification of sewer systems. Home sanitary services were improved, thanks to the water closet which had been invented at the end of the 18th century. Paris set the example in the management of residual waters. During the time of Napoleon, the first underground sewage drains were constructed in Paris. A commendable project, but insufficient to resolve the problem.

It Looks Good On Paper, But...

It is interesting to note that it was more than 1700 years ago that the first agreements were made in regard to environmental protection, and more than 200 years ago that governments dedicated large sums of money and effort to the cause. On paper, our world finds itself fully and completely protected. International laws exist that are designed to conserve the environment. Some 170 treaties that have been ratified within the last 20 years have environmental stipulations; such as: the quantity of fish that may be caught, how many trees may be felled, how much toxic waste may be dispersed in a given region and which species of animal shall be protected. But this paradise only exists in filed documents within the political machinery of international diplomacy. In other words, the coverage of these treaties is as good as the coverage of the back side of a hospital gown!

Private industry is difficult to regulate but governments should be able to control their own industrial giants. However, they often fail to do so. An example of this is the case of the military industrial complex of the United States, which discards 400,000 tons of liquid toxic waste annually. Between 1950 and 1990, 74 million tons of toxic mercury were introduced into the environment. According to government regulations, this residue is three thousand times higher than the accepted level. Such toxicity has staggering repercussions on our world. In Japan many children have been born with congenital deformities because the mothers ate mercury contaminated fish. Yet, nothing has been done to significantly rectify the problem.

Ecological movements have sought to restore the balance between humans and the environment, but the efforts have been half-hearted and they have not been effective in preserving our ecosystem. For example, in the United States, a pact for the preservation of sea mammals was ratified which imposed severe sanctions on fisherman who kill dolphins. In October of 1991 and then in May of 1994, the United States requested an embargo on the importation of Mexican tuna because Mexican fishermen were killing large numbers of dolphins. The request was denied because the embargo conflicted with the rules of GATT, the General Accord on Tariffs and Trade.

Furthermore, the Mexican fishermen alleged that the embargo only served to maintain the high price charged by U.S. fisherman and not to save dolphins. And so, we continue to fight conservation regulations because they affect us economically. In many cases, it seems impossible to apply sanctions on those who don't comply with the regulations. If the most powerful country in the world can't maintain simple ecological treaties with a neighboring country, imagine the difficulty of enforcing multi-international treaties like the World Summit in Rio de Janeiro where more than 100 countries participated. The laudable effort was frustrated. First, because debatable the resolutions favored those with ample resources. Second, sound resolutions were blocked by the poor countries that have no budget to activate the programs.

In the decade of the 70s, some scientists warned that the chlorofluorocarbons, like those which are found in refrigerators and aerosols, were eroding the ozone layer, the blue layer of atmosphere which deflects ultraviolet rays. The ultraviolet rays are a major cause of the increasing incidence of skin cancer in the last few decades, as well as the increase in visual problems. In 1919, it was discovered that a hole had been torn in the ozone 32 miles in diameter over the region of Antarctica. At present, this rip in the ozone layer has grown to equal the size of the United States. The chemical substances responsible for this destruction are used in products such as fire extinguishers and deodorant sprays. Because this alarming trend could endanger the very existence of humanity, the United Nations convened its members to seek some solution.

In 1987, representatives from 140 countries signed an agreement called the *Treaty of Montreal*, in order to protect the ozone layer. This agreement, although well intentioned, left much to be desired. All the countries pledged to prohibit the manufacturing of products containing chlorofluorocarbons (CFC's) by January 1996. In 1988, there were so many products containing CFC's that 1.3 billion kilograms (1.43 million tons) of CFC's had to be produced. Thanks to the Treaty of Montreal, annual production dropped to 510 million kilograms (561 thousand tons) by 1993. Nevertheless, fewer than 80% of the countries involved kept their promise and the goal for reduction was not reached. The penalties imposed on the transgressing countries are insignificant or impossible to exercise. Consequently, the efforts of government authorities who saw the need for action were frustrated.

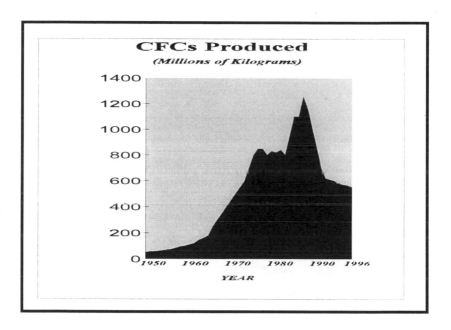

Environmental Diseases

As a result of constantly rising levels of environmental contamination, a new type of modern plague, the environmental disease, has arisen. Some of these diseases are easy to recognize, like cancer, cardiovascular diseases, arthritis, and the explosion of respiratory diseases in large cities. Others have a great variety of manifestations and their diagnosis is complicated.

In general, we lump together environmental diseases that are difficult to identify under the heading of allergies. For example, in Wimberley, Texas, a group of ecologically-challenged people have had to take extreme measures to isolate themselves from the outside world. When someone comes to visit, dialogue can only take place by means of an intercom system. No visitor may enter the waiting room without fulfilling a series of strict requirements. Their clothes must be made from natural fibers and must not contain any dyes. They must be cleaned of any perfume, lotion, soap, and deodorant. They can not bring magazines or newspapers because of the irritant and toxic odor of ink. The list of requirements is endless.

This is not some religious sect nor is it some group of crazy visionaries, but simply sufferers of a 20th century disease which has been called hypersensitivity to chemical substances or environmental disease. According to Delphine Garcia in the magazine *Muy Interesante*, many chemical elements today can cause humans to develop a hypersensitivity to totally natural elements. Consequently, these people are ambushed by contamination that comes from water, air and even common elements within the home.

Don't Drink The Water

Although many of us may not be this sensitive to the myriad of contaminants in the world around us, the contamination of the water supply does threaten to affect all of us. Humanity has always used the seas as a giant natural trash can, believing that the various biological cycles will absorb waste and purify the water. However, we can now prove that in water there exists a balance generated by its chemical, physical and biological elements. The dumping of residual waters in an uncontrolled fashion has converted some coastal regions into an environment where dangerous bacteria thrive. These bacteria threaten the health of the populous, as happened in Italy in 1973 when a harvest of contaminated mussels produced a severe epidemic of cholera.

In the year 1956, a similar and very dramatic case of food poisoning occurred in the region of the Bay of Minamata, Japan. The problem was traced to a factory that dumped untreated waste into the ocean. One hundred and twenty-one people were poisoned when they ate contaminated crustaceans and mollusks. Forty percent of these victims died from cerebral lesions.

A more shocking example took place in 1940 with the birth of the petrochemical industry. Scientists discovered how to produce synthetic products, a discovery which promised to lower costs and introduce thousands of useful products for

consumers. In that year, 1 billion pounds of chemically synthetic substances, which had never been seen in nature before, were produced. During the following decade, production rose to 50 billion pounds and by the 1980s half a trillion
pounds. Obviously it was impossible for governmental agencies to investigate each one of these chemical substances created to determine their level of toxicity.

In the United States, there are 4 million recognized chemical
compoundsses. This number increases each year by approximately 1000 new products. The time and cost of laboratory
tests makes it impossible to keep up with production. Millions of substances have not been tested, yet it is known that
some 600 of them are highly carcinogenic. It took three decades and 40 million dollars to unequivocally prove that tobacco causes cancer. The producers of cigarettes relied on
huge economic resources to counteract these investigations.
Just imagine the vast resources of the petrochemical industry! Meanwhile these chemicals and their byproducts are spoil-
ing the soil and the water.

Impure water has been a problem since the Middle Ages. In
the 19th century, the growth of cities gave rise to such a vast
increase in sewage that nearby fields, wells and rivers were
contaminated. Europe and America tried to solve the problem by creating two separate systems, one to supply
clean water and another to dispose of sewage. Today,
maintenance of these two systems involves some type of

treatment. Tap water is filtered and purified with chlorine, and raw sewage is submitted to one or more treatment processes. Nevertheless, sewage is frequently discharged into canals and oceans without any kind of treatment.

In 1972, the United States initiated a program to build sewage treatment plants throughout the nation. Unfortunately, water treatment plants cannot even detect, much less detoxify, most of the chemical substances that are dumped into the water. Present methods of treatment consist of filtering out dangerous waste from known sources of contaminants. This seems to be a good start but the reality is that new contaminants escape even the most modern filtration systems. A survey of tap water reserves, conducted in 954 U.S. cities, revealed that 30% are contaminated with 17 kinds of very dangerous pesticides.

It is calculated that the chemical industry in the United States produces 60,000 highly toxic compounds that end up in the water supply. The government claims to enforce laws that prohibit the production of many of these substances. However, it is well known that small chemical plants are not effectively monitored and that the industry giants falsify reports and bribe federal agencies. When threatened, some of these companies cover their tracks by criminally disposing of the contaminants into rivers, sewer systems, lakes, and oceans. In this way, they manage to avoid sanctions, fines, and closures. One can only conclude that in Mexico, and other third world countries, the problem is worse for lack of resources and the "laxity" of the government officials.

So, water pollution continues to be the environmental problem that plagues us the most. Paris has a network of drains considered to be one of the most efficient systems on the planet. However, when there is a storm, all the water cannot be treated and excess is discharged into the River Seine without purification. If the most efficient system in the world can't provide complete protection from dangerous toxins, what can we expect from the antiquated and neglected systems in the majority of the world's cities?

Special Waste

In May of 1971, at the Shenandoah Stables in St. Louis, 3,800 liters of oil were spread on the ground to control the dust stirred up in the arena where the horses were trained. This is a common practice in this business. This time however birds, cats, and dogs in the area began to die from dehydration. Of the 85 horses held there to be trained, 43 died within a year. It was not long before the owners of the stables began to suffer headaches, chest pains and severe diarrhea. Several studies were conducted in an effort to find out what was causing this situation. It was discovered that the oil poured on the soil contained dioxin, a highly toxic contaminant. It became apparent that the contaminant had not been removed from the oil before it was applied to the ground. Oil companies are required to remove any toxic materials before selling oil for these purposes. Yet, this illegal and irresponsible act is one of thousands of incidents that take place every day in the world.

Special wastes are substances generated by industry, agriculture or the government that, because of their dangerous nature, must be disposed of in a special or extraordinary way. It is estimated that in the United States of America, a ton of special wastes is produced per person every year by the commercial industry, but the US military industry generates about one ton of toxic waste EVERY MINUTE, from chemical weapons to lethal radioactive materials. Experience has shown that the poor management of special wastes is extremely expensive to correct. In spite of the efforts to adequately control the disposal of these wastes, many countries cannot count on sufficient infrastructure, either administrative or technological, to provide adequate supervision over the final disposal of these materials.

A way must be found to properly dispose of the thousands of tons of toxic sediments that filter out in industrial discharges. Deep burial has been the preferred method for disposing of special waste, especially radioactive material, due to their extreme hazard. In this process wastes are deposited in hermetically sealed containers before burial in the ground. Yet, it is impossible to avoid leaking these poisons into the soil and water sources over time. It is equally difficult to prevent a significant portion of them from being intentionally poured out in streams, rivers and seas.

It is estimated that a cup and a half of contaminated liquid per hour can contaminate 3.8 million liters of water within a day.

In the United States, toxic residues are simply driven to one of over 300,000 official storage sites. But in Mexico and many other countries, there is a very limited capacity for adequately attending to the problem of special wastes. In 1993, Mexico proudly reported that there were 42 companies licensed in Mexico for the management, treatment and disposal of special wastes. The financial resources of Mexico (not of its politicians) is infinitely smaller than those of the US, but to rely on only 42 official depositories is ridiculous. In the eye of many countries, Mexico is a rich nation. Enormous quantities of these materials end up in ordinary dumps. No place is far enough away for these noxious wastes!

In America, it is calculated that many toxic materials are stored in some 50,000 clandestine warehouses. The government is aware of their existence but these warehouses are not closed down because the legal waste sites can not handle the volume of toxic materials produced.

Note that in America the incidence of environmental disease is much higher in urban areas near stockpiles of toxic materials. The Environmental Protection Agency reported that in 240 counties studied, the incidence of breast cancer was significantly higher in counties that contain nuclear facilities or radioactive waste dumps. Why do African-Americans suffer a higher incidence of cancer? One might think that they have a weaker immune system, but in other parts of the world, that race does not show as high an incidence of cancer. In 1987, a study was published entitled "Toxic Waste and Race in the United States and North America" in which the government was accused of placing dumps for toxic and high risk materials in areas strongly populated by African-Americans. In 1993, the Center for Political Alternatives reported that the situation had grown even more serious.

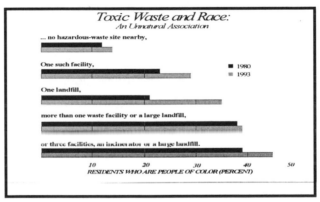

The graph clearly demonstrates that Caucasians have less chance of being exposed to the dangerous effects of these poisons. Obviously these waste sites are installed in places where land is cheaper, but it is possible that government agencies also count on the lack of resistance from the lower socioeconomic population. Consequently, the incidence of cancer and other environmental diseases is very high for these people.

Furthermore, many companies travel to other countries to illegally dump these deadly materials. At the World Summit in Rio and in the ecological Convention in Basel, Switzerland, activists and governmental officials insisted that these toxic materials be disposed of in the places where they are produced, except for those materials that can't be environmentally managed in the countries of origin. This is not only fair, but the risk of accidents taking place during transport is eliminated. Wealthy countries aren't wild about having to wash their dirty laundry at home, nevertheless, 22 Latin-American and Caribbean countries do not permit their soil to be used as toxic landfills and African nations are following suit.

Nature can't keep up. Its water processing capability is insufficient to supply the enormous worldwide demand; so our rivers, subterranean springs, lakes, reservoirs and oceans are swarming with these venomous manmade substances.

The Air We Breathe

In our world today, it is becoming increasingly difficult to step outside to get a breath of "fresh air." The industrialized world around us pours tons of sulfur dioxide and other toxic substances into the air each day. Naturally, as we go about our lives, we don't think about the toxic gases in the air we breath. Yet, we know that these toxins undermine the health of the populous because every day we hear more about pulmonary diseases, allergies and fatigue.

In 1990, the government of Mexico City revealed that its steadily increasing air pollution was seriously jeopardizing the health of the city's inhabitants. Some 13,500 tons of contaminants were being produced there each day, the most of any city in the world. A frightful figure if you consider that the environmental agency is very concerned because 74,000 tons are produced daily in the *whole* US, with hundreds of industrialized cities. Unless firm measures are taken, it is estimated that by the year 2000, the level of worldwide contamination will double.

he invention of the wheel changed the course of history, but it was the gasoline motors that caused the most commotion. With the invention of the automobile, high speed transportation became a reality. One way or another, we depend on this invention. The toxic product linked to gasoline that is the most dangerous is lead. This heavy metal has a powerful negative affect on our health. In Mexico City, 20,000 infants are born every year with lead in the bloodstream. In the nation as a whole, 7.7 million children have been affected by this toxic agent, according to the National Institute of Public Health. The principle access route of lead into our bodies is through the air we breathe, but we all ingest between 1000 and 2000 micrograms of lead from the processed foods we eat every day. Not surprisingly, 74% of children from populated cities have critically high concentrations of lead in their blood.

Experts in the field agree that the human body should be 100% free of this metal. Lead poisoning can cause brain lesions, neuropsychological dysfunction, behavior problems, mental retardation, kidney problems and death.

Thousands of other toxic elements are introduced into the air from motors, petroleum refineries, the chimneys of the chemical industry, etc. This filthy soup is known as smog. In 1930 in a Belgian city, 60 people died because of smog and 60,000 became ill for the same reason. In London, 40,000 people died and hundreds of thousands were affected by smog in 1952. I could find no statistics about this problem for Mexico City, I believe they are too alarming to be published and our country is not prepared for such panic. Smog is a product of hydrocarbon, nitrous oxide, and other particles that, upon being exposed to sunlight, become toxic. Although in some countries like Japan, Germany and the United States, standards have been established to control toxic emissions, in many other developing countries, no substantive change is foreseen in the near future.

The main source of the toxic emissions which give rise to smog are motorized vehicles. A study by the University of Southern California demonstrates the damage done by smog. Researchers performed autopsies on 100 young auto accident victims from the Los Angeles area. They found that there was severe smog related damage to the lungs of all these young people. The chief researcher stated that young people who live in large cities are literally having their lungs destroyed. Our organism is not designed to expel smog particles. Thankfully, some of the toxins are eliminated by the kidneys. Unfortunately, the smog particles that are not eliminated often pass into the bloodstream and accumulate in fatty tissue and other cells. This causes all kinds of damage, often irreversible, not only to humans but to animals and plants.

Air pollution gets worse in the winter because smog remains trapped in the warm surface air and becomes concentrated and more toxic. This phenomenon has been called thermal inversion. In Mexico City, thermal inversion has been so acute that schools have been closed in the month of December. Mexico City is home to the most important economic, political and cultural activities of the Mexican nation. It is home to one-fifth of the national population, some 20 million people. It is also home to 3 million motor vehicles, 30,000 industrial enterprises, and 12,000 service enterprises. The city is cursed with certain geographical characteristics which make it difficult to disperse smog. It is equally cursed with certain meteorological conditions which aggravate the problem.

The illnesses traced to this pollution include difficulty breathing, vertigo, headaches, laryngitis, eye irritation, nausea, asthma, bronchitis, pulmonary emphysema, pneumonia, lung cancer, vascular diseases, skin diseases, reduction of red blood cells, lead damage to kidneys, mental retardation, sterility, and high risk pregnancies. The people of Mexico City are most at risk during periods of thermal inversion, which occur around 180 days per year and last about five hours. In 1940 the visibility in Mexico City was 10 miles, now it is less than 2. To improve these conditions, the "Integrated Program Against Atmospheric Contamination" was initiated in 1990. This plan was to implement 42 specific projects designed to address the problem of air pollution in Mexico City. However, the fact remains that Mexico doesn't have the money to implement it nor the infrastructure. Efforts to decentralize its capital have been futile, so there isn't much hope that such programs will prosper in the near future. For instance, a program to diminish the circulation of autos by 20% was put into effect by limiting their use to 6 days a week. The cars are grounded one day of the week depending on the last number or letter of the license plate. Brilliant idea, but the government did not supply the mass transportation needed and the citizens went and bought cars with different license plates. The only ones who benefited were the used car salesman! Smog concentration has reached such a level that, occasionally, the city has literally been shut down by closing all factories and only allowing 50% of official vehicles to circulate.

All large cities have too much smog. Entrepreneurs in New York have come up with an interesting idea to help citizens cope with the poor air quality. They opened the "oxygen bar," where, for the price of an expensive cup of coffee, you will get a little hose with two small tubes you place in your nostrils for 20 minutes to inhale 100% oxygen. Only in America!

The Earth's Lungs

Nature depends on trees to metabolize toxic agents and cleanse the air. This system is very effective but the original design cannot handle the astronomical quantities of contaminants we produce.

The frailty of our intelligence is exposed when, in addition to polluting our world, we complicate nature's work through the exploitation of natural resources, especially deforestation by the lumber industry. Winds, drought, hurricanes, twisters and other climatic factors as well as indiscriminate urban and industrial growth and soil contamination contribute to the waning forests.

In our world, less than 55% of the forests remain intact. This has contributed to the reduction of oxygen in the atmosphere. If deforestation continues at its present rate, 4% of the earth's surface per year, there will be no forests left by the year 2035. There is genuine worldwide concern about deforestation because trees play a crucial role in the cleaning of our air supply. The fact is that there is no simple solution to the series of problems related to atmospheric pollution but scientists and ecologists are diligently working. In Germany, a forest lab has been created in Solling near the river Weser where they are "teaching" trees to live with pollution. China has planted trees in more than 500, 000 acres. Iceland, in celebration of its 50 years of independence, has allocated one billion dollars in reforestation. The Mexican government gives trees to any one who will plant them and the response has been excellent.

But technological advances have added a new type of air contamination, radio frequencies and electromagnetic fields. Employees of electrical companies have a significantly higher rate of cancer due to exposure to high voltage and high tech instrumentation. In San Diego, California birds are flying disoriented because of the numerous Magnetic Resonance Imaging machines (a type of x-ray without x-rays) where the images are produced by an enormous magnet.

Acid Rain

Rain, blessing or curse? "Good morning" Said the weatherman of a radio station in Los Angeles, California… "the satellite shows a possibility of 80% of *acid* rain today, take your umbrella and may God be with you!"

Precipitation made up of water and contaminants, especially sulfuric oxide and nitrous oxide which are catalyzed in the atmosphere and dropped to the earth, is called acid rain.

The contaminants can also be precipitated with snow or dust clouds. Let's remind ourselves that the United States expels more than 74,000 tons of sulfuric dioxide into the atmosphere every day and that this is only one of the thousands of impurities introduced into the air each day. Others are nitrous oxide, hydrocarbons, carbon monoxide, lead, and the well known fluorocarbons, the destroyers of the ozone layer. The effect of acid rain on plants, seas, lakes and rivers, not to mention humans, is incredible. It is responsible for wiping out the marine life in several lakes in Canada as well as some in Europe. From now on the old children's song should be sung like this: "It's raining, it's pouring, the old man is snoring. It's acid rain, smog to blame, he shouldn't get up this morning!"

Is It Hot In Here, Or What?

In Germany, thousands of acres of the black forest have been destroyed and more than 100,000 acres have been damaged from the "greenhouse effect," or global warming. The massive amounts of carbon dioxide introduced into our atmosphere each day absorbs the ultraviolet light of the sun and holds in the heat, thus raising the environmental temperature. We were warned that global warming would occur if we continued polluting the air with carbon dioxide (at a rate of 5 billion metric tons per year). Scientists predict that the polar ice caps will melt, elevating sea levels by 18 feet, and that fields that are now fertile will be converted into deserts. Is there no end to the environmental disasters that loom over us?

Other Problems of Contamination

There are a host of dangerous toxins we have ignored. These fall into four categories:

- Synthetic organic chemicals like benzene and many pesticides
- Natural chemical substances like chlorine, ammonia and hydrogen fluoride
- Toxic fibers like carcinogenic asbestos
- Toxic metals like mercury, nickel and cadmium

It is impossible for any government to do tests on each of the millions of synthetic organic chemicals produced by industry. If a substance is tested and proven harmful, its production may be banned. On the rare occasions that the law is applied, it only serves as a "Band-Aid" cure because the industry giants merely seek out some third world country that, because of employment opportunities and the occasional bribe, will allow them to manufacture such poisonous products. I'm not absolving the poor, but it is a major sin that civilized men would use such a strategy to avoid regulations designed to protect people's lives. The consequences often are disastrous. On December 3, 1984, a damaged tank belonging to Union Carbide, a US transnational company established in Bhopal, India, began to leak a poisonous gas.

This leak caused the death of 3,500 inhabitants and injured 200,000 more. The government of India filed a suit in which it charged that Union Carbide had built a plant with architectural defects and that it was not carrying out adequate maintenance. The company alleged that the accident was the product of an act of sabotage by an employee. Finally, in 1989, the U.S. Supreme Court ruled against Union Carbide, and demanded that restitution be made in the amount of 470 million dollars to the survivors. The money has yet to be distributed.

Nuclear Contamination

Radioactive particles introduced into the environment from nuclear explosions and nuclear power plants have worried physicists for decades. Communities in the United States have complained about the amount of nuclear tests performed in the deserts of Nevada and Utah since 1950. For many years, there has been evidence that it is dangerous to become exposed to the residue of such detonations. Yet, no remedial action was undertaken by the United States government until 1984 when a federal judge in Utah ruled that ten people had developed cancer as a result of the radiation produced by military testing. One year later, British courts held their military industry responsible for the elevated incidence of cancer in veterans who had taken part in the testing of nuclear arms at Christmas Island in 1950. Governments have placed a lot of emphasis on protecting the environment from nuclear contamination, and the developed countries have budgeted enormous amounts for this purpose. Yet, contamination of the world's water by nuclear elements is ever increasing. For example, from the industrial county of Love Canal, where one of the largest dumps of nuclear waste is found, comes the following report:

1. The rate of involuntary abortion is three times that of the national average.

2. Fifty-six percent of the county's children suf fer from both physical and mental deficiencies.

3. The incidence of cancer is three times greater than the rest of the country.

In 1970, the community of Love Canal near Niagara Falls had to be evacuated because of a leak of highly toxic radioactive material. The majority of the nation's nuclear waste dumps had been maintained in virtual secrecy but the accident drew attention to them. Countries that handle nuclear materials aren't careful enough in the way in which they dispose of radioactive waste. When the regulations for disposal become too stringent in their own country, they seek to dump waste in other countries that have no experience in handling these dangerous materials; and don't forget the devastating risks of accidents en route. At this moment, the U.S. is building three nuclear dump sites along the border with Mexico. This could prove to be fatal for many living in those areas.

Before the disintegration of the Iron Curtain the world lived under a cloud of fear from a nuclear holocaust. Americans, and thus the rest of the free world, harvested angst because at any moment the Russians, as in a James Bond movie, would press the dreaded "red" button blowing up the world. Many would be pulverized immediately and the rest would die from the agonizing side effects of radiation, envying those who were wiped out. Ironically, the enemy was not on the other side of the ocean. HBO reported that more than 1000 Atomic bombs have been detonated on American soil in military tests. The toxic effects of this volume of testing is staggering.

After an explosion, the atoms of uranium and plutonium produce around 300 radioactive isotopes. This radioactive conglomerate is trapped in the atmosphere and descends slowly to the ground in a radioactive rain. All creatures, especially human, are very sensitive to radioisotopes which invade our bodies through the air, water, and contaminated foods. Even though some of them are fleeting, most will stay in the earth for ever, for instance, the average life of carbon 14 is 5760 years!

On April 26, 1986 in Chernobyl, Ukraine, the world was shaken by the worst nuclear industrial accident in history. The explosion contaminated the atmosphere with 100 million curies of radioisotopes that expanded from the Ukraine to Great Britain. Only 31 people died in the explosion, but to attempt to calculate the total deaths from the radiation introduced into the environment from the accident would be imposible.

Ten thousand deer had to be sacrificed in Europe because they ate contaminated feed from the radioactive rain that will remain for at least 30 years. The problem is not that the Europeans will be deprived of this delicacy, but that they also were bathed with this rain as well as all their crop and soil. The effects will linger for decades because long-term exposure to small doses of radiation can cause serious illness. One of the contaminants was the well known strontium 90, this isotope has been widely researched because it easily contaminates milk. In cases where animals or humans are exposed to it, the incidence of leukemia and cancer of the bone is significantly higher than the rest of the population.

Mormons have enjoyed a low incidence of cancer because they avoid the consumption of caffeine, alcohol and tobacco. Ironically, the incidence of cancer has increased among them because many of them live in Utah, close to atomic test sites. Victims of Hiroshima and Nagasaki have an extraordinarily high rate of cancer, but malignancies are not the only risk; they also suffer from small skulls and brains thus functionally impaired.

One of the most threatening risks of radiation is that of mutations. Remember that hereditary information is found in the genes. Almost all radioactive materials can induce genetic mutations. Before protection against radiation was so sophisticated, tests were made on the families of 2000 radiologists. Tests revealed that the index of fetal deaths was higher than in the rest of the population, and congenital deformities were more frequent than in the children of doctors in other specialties. In addition, changes in the morphology of the sperm of radiologists and specialists in nuclear medicine have also been observed, even when protective measures were taken. There are no safe levels of radiation.

Activists want nuclear energy plants to be dismantled for the threat they are to our world. But the fact is that half of the radiation we normally receive comes from the sun and natural isotopes that exist in the water, soil and atmosphere. The other half is manmade: 10% by the nuclear plants and 90% from the medical industry (x-rays, nuclear medicine and radiation therapy). Who will protect us from the doctors?

Domestic Garbage

Now let's talk about a more mundane but no less disturbing topic - domestic trash. Dumps throughout the world are bulging. Taking into account the fact that the average city dweller produces a half ton of garbage every year, it is obvious that disposal space is limited. The exasperating thing is that about 90% of the volume of trash is reducible, providing people do the following three things:

1. Remove empty spaces (flattening boxes, mashing cans, etc.).
2. Compost biodegradable materials.

3. Recycle what can be reused (glass, plastics, paper, etc.).

American citizens produce the largest amounts of domestic waste among the developed, "throw away society," countries.

Country	Annual Domestic Waste (Tons)	Equivalent per person (Kilograms)
Australia	10,000,000	680
Belgium	3,082,000	313
Canada	12,600,000	525
Denmark	2,046,000	399
Finland	1,200,000	399
France	15,500,000	288
Great Britain	15,816,000	282
Italy	14,041,000	246
Japan	40,225,000	288
Netherlands	5,400,000	381
New Zealand	1,528,000	488
Norway	1,700,000	415
Spain	8,028,000	214
Sweden	2,500,000	300
Switzerland	2,146,000	336
United States	200,000,000	875
West Germany	20,780,000	337

Source: World Health Organization

These countries have adopted ample recycling programs to separate the reusable components from the trash. Furthermore, the designated dumping sites in these countries are quite capable of handling trash adequately. The following is a list of the quantities of domestic trash by country and per person in some of the more developed countries.

Recycling

In France, special recycling machines have been installed in many supermarkets. When a person recycles aluminum cans the machine gives out bonds to purchase merchandise. The purpose is to create incentive and consciousness in consumers so that they will cooperate in the recycling effort. In Mexico City, 100 schools participate in a contest to collect the most waste paper. The paper is sold and the proceeds fund other programs that teach children the importance of recycling. An interesting program is the one implemented by the National Center for Environmental Education and the Mexican Ecological Movement. This program provides educational materials to 10,000 teachers and 640,000 students. In exchange, the schools agree to carry out campaigns that promote decontamination, civic neatness, and recycling. Yet, isolated efforts like these don't adequately address the worldwide problem.

Composting

One method of disposing garbage is called composting, a process in which organic garbage is transformed into a fertilized soil called compost. In this process, inorganic trash (rags, glass, cans, scrap metal, plastics, cardboard, paper, wood, bones, etc.) must be separated from the organic. The organic garbage becomes compost through a process of bacterial fermentation, which destroys the toxic elements present in raw garbage. The use of compost for agricultural purposes has been practiced in many countries for a long time. Besides fertilizing the soil, compost improves it physically in terms of its texture and structure. Its use on diverse kinds of cultivated crops has yielded highly satisfactory results on the harvest. Compost also has a high capacity for retaining water which might otherwise erode soil. Compost offers the following benefits:

1. Betters the structure and texture of soil.
2. Increases the capacity of soil to retainmoisture.
3. Helps avoid flood damage in the rainy season and cracking in the drought season.
4. Facilitates field work like plowing, weeding, etc.
5. Enriches the ground with organic material: humus, minerals and microorganisms. These are highly beneficial to the development of vegetation.
6. Releases nutrients slowly so nothing is wasted.
7. Provokes the freeing of nutrients found in the mineral segments of the soils.
8. Increases harvest production and the material earnings per acre.
9. Contains no photogenic microorganisms.

European countries have industrialized compost production since 1942. In Mexico and other countries, attempts havebeen made, but without much success because this industry requires specialized machinery and trained personnel, as well as a huge initial investment of capital. But home composting is easy and cheap. Any hardware store will give you information on how to do it.

Indoor Pollution

To avoid smog, people stay in enclosed places. However, enclosed spaces aren't free from pollution either. In the United States, office workers frequently suffer from unexplainable irritation of the eyes and skin. When customers and employees of a bank in Encino, California, experienced headaches, nausea and vomiting, officials determined that the cause was excessive concentration of carbon monoxide, 20 times more than the concentration accepted in smog contaminated air! In the future it is possible that indoor contamination could become a greater problem than external contamination. Allergist, Dr. Alfred Zamm, discovered that the air inside the typical American home contains "carbon monoxide, nitric acid, and nitrogen dioxide in concentrations up to four times the maximum accepted by federal guidelines."

Las Vegas casinos provide, among other luxuries, high tech air. Cleansed and oxygenated with ozone which invigorates patrons and keeps them awake. Of course the health of clients is "why" they made the investment, the fact that they spend more time throwing their money into the slot machines was unexpected! We should all ozonify our houses and offices; fortunately, these machines are becoming easier to acquire.

Our homes often lack adequate ventilation so that pure air is limited and harmful elements can reach very high levels. The danger represented by indoor contaminants is aggravated by the lack of information about the problem. The best known contaminants are asbestos, formaldehyde and lead.

Asbestos is highly prized for its cost effectiveness and resistance to heat. Almost all buildings have asbestos, particularly schools. In the US about 15 million children are exposed to it and yet, it is a proven cause of asbestosis, malignant mesothelioma, lung, mouth, larynx, esophagus, stomach, kidney and colon cancer. Developed countries have started to abandon the use of this material. Too late for the 11 million people who will die from cancer caused by asbestos products.

Formaldehyde toxins are present in certain textiles, plywood, rugs, and molded plastics. They are also found in deodorants, shampoos, hair conditioners, tooth paste, mouthwash, detergents and room deodorizers. These chemicals are highly allergenic and more and more people are becoming extremely sensitive to them.

We have already spoken of the contamination of the air by lead (smog). Yet, there is some additional information that may be useful. Lead is also found in water pipes, plastics, ceramic containers, and products painted with oil paints. Children are very susceptible to lead poisoning. The symptoms of lead poisoning are stomach ache, constipation, vomiting, hyperactivity, diminishing IQ, aggressive behavior, attention deficit disorder, impaired vision, impaired hearing, slow reaction time, slow growth, and poor balance. Too often doctors misdiagnose children and give the wrong treatment. In 1992, the Secretary of Health and Human Services in the United States declared, lead poisoning to be the most common environmental sickness and socially it is the most devastating among small children. Mexican researchers have come to the conclusion that 25% of the children have lead poisoning, resulting in an alarming high rate of learning disabilities and low IQ levels. In Paris, hundreds of children are hospitalized annually by lead poisoning. Of 600 children treated, 200 suffered considerable brain damage. Dr. Yves Manuel, toxicologist and advisor to the French Ministry of Ecology, stated that the children throughout the country were in danger of suffering irreversible brain damage.

Experts calculate that we are in constant contact with some 34,000 highly toxic manmade products that our body cannot metabolize or neutralize. The threat is real because many of these products are found within the confines of our own homes, schools, churches, theaters, stores and offices. We must collectively decide to do something to protect ourselves.

Measures To Counteract The Ecological Disaster

In the face of the prevailing conditions on the planet, a United Nations Conference, better known as the "World Summit," was held in Rio de Janeiro, Brazil, to establish international treaties designed to protect the environment. Some of the principles proclaimed were:

Principle 7: Various countries should cooperate with a spirit of world solidarity, protecting and re-establishing the health and integrity of the world's ecosystem. In view of the fact that all have been contributing in varying degrees to the destruction of world environment, the governments have common responsibilities.

Principle 11: Countries should enact effective laws relating to the environment.

Principle 14: Countries should discourage or avoid the relocation and transfer to other countries of substances that cause serious environmental degradation or that are considered dangerous to human health.

Principle 16: National authorities should strive to promote the internationalization of environmental costs and the use of economic instruments, taking into account the criteria that those who pollute should bear the cost of the contamination, keeping also in mind public interest and the avoidance of distorting trade or international investments.

Principle 19: Countries should give out pertinent information to those states that can be affected by disposal activities that could have substantial noxious impact on environments across borders.

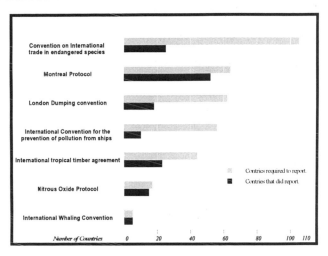

These principles seem to mark the beginning of a process
that could solve the ecological problem. Or do they? The
intended world solidarity stated in Principle 7 was violated in
the same conference. The United States, China, and OPEC
strongly opposed any attempt to regulate toxic gas emissions
in favor of greater energy efficiency, despite the overwhelming evidence that toxic gases are the major cause
of acid rain and other ecological disasters. Prior to the conference, the effort was made toward the conservation of
forests with legal force included, but this effort was frustrated, principally by Malaysia. Malaysia possesses one of
the largest extensions of forests and has been accused of
excessive deforestation. The following graph reveals the
goodwill inherent in some of the agreements signed by

multiple nations and the sad reality of the few that keep their vows.

Why don't we stop? Are we crazy? The following example suggests that we just might be. A copper smelter in Tacoma, WA, contaminates the atmosphere with arsenic, causing 2 deaths per year for each 100 inhabitants. The government proposed to close the plant, putting 575 families out of work. The closing of the plant was put to a vote among the inhabitants. For practical purposes, round off the population of Tacoma to 100,000 people. This means that 2000 inhabitants per year will die of arsenic poisoning or 20 persons for each 1000 inhabitants. In the United States, the number one cause of death is cardiovascular disease, which kills 1 million people out of a population of 250 million, or 4 people for each 1000 inhabitants. The incidence of death from the arsenic contamination in Tacoma is five times the number one cause of death in the United States. Yet, the inhabitants voted to keep the factory open. That is insanity.

Still, there is always someone who will give an example to emulate. I want to tell you of an experience in contrast to the Tacoma case. At the base of the Matterhorn is one of the most beautiful panoramas in Switzerland and the entire world. It is one of those places that makes you gasp in awe when you see it. It is visited by painters, poets, writers, skiers, mountain climbers and tourists from all over the world. When my family and I had a chance to visit the Matterhorn, I didn't doubt for a moment that we would go.

We took the automobile trip with some friends, but the highway ended a long way before we arrived at the famous mountain. We had to park the car and board an electric train. This seemed a major inconvenience to me especially when you travel with small children. However, it was explained to me that the inhabitants of the region pledged to protect the purity of the environment, so gas and diesel motorized vehicles weren't allowed. To get around, the local residents travel by foot, bicycle, horseback, and electric carts in case of emergency. The inconvenience does scare away many tourists. Yet, the residents of the region have chosen alternatives that reveal love and respect for their descendants and for nature, even at the expense of their economy.

Thank God for people like that. I have a friend, Virginia Setzer (friends call her Ginny), that has great respect and love for our world. Preoccupied about the environmental impact of domestic waste, she decided that her household was not going to contribute to the problem and began separating garbage, recycling and composting. Mind you, this was a foreign concept in Guadalajara, Mexico, where she lived at the time. Soon she found out that it was not complicated and she began to get her neighbors involved too. Slowly her influence grew and in 1990 she was awarded a prize for her activities by her gardening club. Other associations and schools started to invite her to speak about recycling

Alejandro Juarez from the local newspaper reported that more than 15,000 households were trained to separate and recycle through her teachings (Oct. 13,1994). The city responded by establishing centers to receive the separated wastes. She has organized her neighbors to work for the environment and along with 100 ecologists, they planted 65,000 trees. As a reward for her efforts, the community officials named the reforested area "Ginny's Woods."

Each of us can demonstrate the same attitude in our immediate surroundings. We don't have to be a member of the government or belong to some ecological institution. We can begin to take care of our environment in our own home and neighborhood. It is a matter of contributing at the level of our resources and demonstrating our commitment to ourselves and our children. As Alfred Lord Tennyson, "Man is man, an architect of his own destiny." Yes, we have to go back to nature to secure our future.

Chapter 3

Hunger Is Vicious

There is no more sincere love than the love of food.

George Bernard Shaw

The Food Industry

Humans can't live long without eating. Even under normal conditions, most humans find it uncomfortable to experience hunger for even a few minutes. It is possible, under extreme circumstances, to live a few weeks without food. However, when reserved calories stored in the fat and muscles are consumed, death soon follows.

The Mexican saying, "hunger is vicious," truly depicts human nature and the desperate tendencies hunger can bring out in us. My country, Mexico, is going through a political turmoil which is devastating the economy leaving millions without work. Many bread winners have little choice but to steal in order to provide food for their families. When circumstances become extreme, even civilized people have been driven to cannibalism. Who can forget the gruesome story of the Donner party and more recently, as depicted in the movie "Alive," the young athletes who suffered the same food deprivation after their plane crashed in the High Andes? Sheer desperation caused by famine drove thousands to drown themselves in the waters of the Tiber river in Rome in 436 BC.

The majority of historians record some 400 famines. The worst of these took place in India in 769 when 10 million people died, and in China when a similar number died in 1877. In the 20th century around 4 million Chinese paid the ultimate price of hunger in the Province of Henan.

Until the end of the 19th century, the majority of human beings lived on a very restricted and monotonous diet, dependent on what the land produced in each region and on the seasons of the year. Food was cultivated, gathered, cooked and eaten. The Industrial Revolution brought aboutincreased food production and new methods of preservation. Currently, the US alone produces more food than is needed for all the inhabitants of the world. Yet, we continue to experience famine. Why? Wars, droughts, floods and other natural factors ruin foodstuffs, but the ugly reality is that politics and economics are the true assassins. Food is either destroyed or stored to maintain its high market value so that even when it's available, many around the globe, in rich and poor countries, cannot afford to eat.

Moliere, a French philanthropist said three centuries ago, "One should eat to live not live to eat." While for many food is out of reach, the ones that have means overeat and waste it. Still, most likely, we are undernourished in spite of our "love handles." The Industrial Revolution gave birth to an industry that has mechanized, electrified, fertilized, pesticized, sterilized, refined, and processed foodstuffs. Food production exploded (as well as our waists and thighs) with an inversely proportional nutritional value.

Years ago, we produced food to survive; now we produce food to make money. Modern agriculture has become a lucrative industry which is forever on the lookout for ways to become even more profitable. One doesn't need to search very far to discover how increased productivity affects profit in the food business. Many increase productivity by manipulating nature with chemical fertilizers to shorten the harvest time, and pesticides to diminish losses. Others increase profit by distributing the product at a time when the best prices can be obtained. However, most industry giants will agree that the best way to increase profit is to transform perishable food into non-perishable food. What is frightening is the fact that the very methods used to increase productivity and profit also severely damage the nutritional value of the food produced. In many cases, the nutritional value is virtually erased.

The mission of the modern food industry is to increase the demand of the foods that bring in the highest profits (Kellogg spends 34 million dollars a year just to promote its frosted flakes: GRRREAT!). Foods are processed to be tasty, precooked and imperishable (indestructible), in other words, they can conveniently stay in your refrigerator or storage forever, and when you want them, a couple of minutes in the "micro" and *viola*! These "high-profit" foods, the backbone of the food industry, are so unnatural and un-nutritional that they represent an authentic health risk. But in this time and age where time is going faster than ever, spending it in the kitchen seems to break all the rules of a politically correct time manager. The fastest growing companies within the food industry are fast (processed, precooked) food corporations. Every eight hours, somewhere in the world, a new fast food restaurant is opened.

Hunger of the affluent society is tastefully, conveniently and artificially quenched by the food industry; unfortunately our bodies need real and nutritious food to meet the challenges of modern existence. Contrary to popular belief, eating is not just a recreational activity. Most people don't spend a great deal of time considering the nutritional quality of the foods they consume. For many individuals, this can prove to be a fatal mistake. Isn't it ironic how fast food, designed to save minutes in our day, ultimately steals years from our lives? Know your foods!

Fruits and Vegetables

You don't have to be a Ph.D. in Nutrition to understand that eating has a more important task than to satisfy hunger. We know intuitively that we have to refuel our bodies with energy. Isn't it interesting that ancient cultures from all parts of the world provide all nutrients necessary to maintain health regardless of the fact that their diets and recipes are so different? According to availability and preferences, cultures have developed their own culinary art, and each recipe is a treaty in biochemistry. Frankly, I doubt that our ancestors spent much time considering the biochemical reactions produced in their rudimentary kitchens, but somehow they knew what was needed and what satisfied requirements and taste buds. Who hasn't "heard" the body tell you that you "need" a hot broth (Jewish penicillin) and rest because of a flu? Yet, it is so easy to forget that the foods we eat are a vehicle for transporting the nutrients that generate the energy our bodies require.

It is just as easy to overlook the fact that almost all nutrients come from the ground. The easiest way to transport nutrients from the soil to our bodies is consuming fruits and vegetables. It's that simple. However, these fresh, perishable foods are quite liable to attacks from a whole variety of natural events from microorganisms to decomposition that threatens the rentability of the business.

Microorganisms have always been a big concern for the industry. War against them is wedged furiously with all kinds of pesticides in order to "protect" the consumer; the truth is that they are protecting their crop from being eaten by the bugs, which, if we wash carefully and cook before we eat the fruits and vegetables, are easily eliminated. To grow the vegetables and fruits bigger and faster, indiscriminate amounts of fertilizers are dumped into the soil and as soon as the harvest is done, the soil is prepared for the next crop. Abuse of our soil and the excessive use of fertilizers and pesticides erodes and strips it of its nutrients. Consequently, the nutritional value of the fruits and vegetables produced from such soil is dramatically diminished. According to the 1980 reference book, *Applied Soil Elements,* published by John Wiley & Sonstrace, trace elements, including boron, chromium, copper, molybdenum, selenium, and zinc, are not found in sufficient quantities in crop plants across much of the USA.

A government study revels that 99% of the American population is mineral deficient. Soil in at least 30 states have been shown to be seriously depleted of zinc. This has resulted because of intensive chemical farming during the past few decades. Surveys recently conducted, over a five year period by West Virginia University, show that the contents of iron, copper and manganese have dropped in grain in 11 Midwestern states. We cannot recur to ignorance; Moses gave us instructions on how to treat our soil in 1490 BC.!

> Six years thou shalt sow thy field, and six years thou shalt prune thy vineyard, and gather in the fruit thereof; But in the seventh year shall be a sabbath of rest unto the land, a sabbath for the LORD: thou shalt neither sow thy field, nor prune thy vineyard. That which groweth of its own accord of thy harvest thou shalt not reap, neither gather the grapes of thy vine undressed: [for] it is a year of rest unto the land.

The most frequently used fertilizers destroy iron, vitamin C, folic acid, minerals, lysine and many other amino acids, among other nutrients. Pesticides contaminate the soil, and take a long time to disappear. For example, chlorodine has a half-life of twenty years. Remember that all plants absorb the substances found in the earth. It does not take much thought to realize that it is downright dangerous to eat fruits and vegetables that contain industrial chemicals. While authorities have prohibited the use of some strong carcinogenic pesticides, the weak carcinogenic pesticides are considered safe (only by a scientist paid by the pesticide industry!). The problem is that in the laboratories they are tested individually. In real life they are always used in combinations because of their synergistic effects which also increases their carcinogenic potential 1000 fold. Also, they forget to tell us that non-carcinogenic pesticides can cause depression, migraines, hyperactivity, etc. Pesticides are easily absorbed and hard to eliminate; they remain in our body with embarrassingly dire consequences because of their chemical affinity to estrogen. I will expound on this subject in the next section.

It's frightening to think that not only produce contain pesticides; the majority (94%) of foods are contaminated with them. Without a doubt, continuous exposure to them can cause cancer and other degenerative diseases. In 1968, a research group found that patients who died from liver cancer, brain cancer, multiple sclerosis and other degenerative diseases, had significantly higher traces of pesticides in their brains and fatty tissue than cadavers who had died from other diseases.

Crushing evidence of pesticide toxicity is forcing the industry to look for new methods of protecting consumers from plagues. This progressive industry has turned to modern age technology and is now using radiation to sanitize produce. Interesting way of protecting us! Radioisotopes not only destroy nutrients, they, as I have already mentioned, are particles that easily enter our cells, increasing the risk of mutation and cancer. The truth is that the public's protection is not the issue; they are protecting their crop.

A few years ago we could only eat certain foods according to the season. Now few foods are ever unavailable. The demands of the consumer and the rentability of the business require efficient management of the soil, harvesting techniques, storage, packaging and transportation of foods. Accelerated produce production in nutrient deprived soil provides handicapped (nutritionally challenged) vegetables and fruits. This leads to physically and mentally challenged human beings.

It is bad enough that the we must eat foods grown in contaminated soil. It's even worse that nutritional value is severely compromised to obtain cosmetic appearance; inexcusable that we must eat them chemically laden. Yet, the average consumer wants to purchase produce that "looks" good. To increase shelf life, farmers harvest their fruits and vegetables long before they are mature, even though it's well established that they absorb most of their vitamins and minerals when they are almost ripe. In order to protect produce from dents, scrapes, and bruises, vegetables and fruits are boxed or piled. Packaging and transportation compromises nutritional value even more. If picked and left outside more than two or three hours, their nutritional value is further reduced 40 to 50 %. In storage, they lose more nutrients. Think about that the next time you pick up a bunch of bright green bananas. They will never fill up with vitamins and minerals sitting on supermarket shelves or on your kitchen counters! Potatoes lose up to 78 % of their vitamin C in a week. Spinach greens, asparagus, broccoli and peas lose 50 % of their vitamins before they ever get to market. However, industrial toxins like aluminum, arsenic, cadmium, nickel, and mercury will remain in us long after we are buried.

"Fresh" produce have the inconvenience of time restriction; processed, they have very long shelf lives and are much more profitable. In addition to toxic fertilizers and pesticides, these life extended vegetables, fruits and their derivatives have other chemicals that further undermine our bodies. Juices and milk are usually packaged in carton containers lined with wax, a known carcinogen. Plastic containers aren't much better since they are made from petrochemicals, polymers with toxic stabilizers and color tinctures like acrylic acid, tuolene, styrofoam and vinyl chloride. These elements abound in disposable plates, bowls and cups and are carcinogens.

Availability and convenience are the forces that move the industry to provide imperishable-user-friendly foods to the consumer in cans or frozen bags, but in every step of the process, they lose even more of the few nutrients left. Frozen vegetables lose 25% of vitamins A, B1, B2, C and niacin among others. Broccoli, cauliflower, peas and spinach lose up to 50% of vitamins. Canned foods lose more than 50% of all nutrients but provide a substantial amount of lead! To avoid botulism nitrites are used ...good. When nitrites are heated (these foods usually are) they are converted into nitrosamines, potent carcinogens ...bad.

By the time these "new tech" foods get to our mouths, they have already been submitted to a vast number of tortures. They have been treated with acidifiers, alkalinizers, anti-foaming agents, artificial colors, artificial flavors, sweeteners, deodorants, fillers, disinfectants, emulsifiers, extenders, hydrogenators, moisturizers and plenty more etceteras. Oh yes, and a good portion of synthetic vitamins! These modern and profitable foods are so well made that they are practically indestructible. Sluggishly, but surely, our organisms are destroyed by them.

With no obstruction from the authorities, backed by major investors, encouraged by the flourishing business and unleashed by our ignorance, food producers force feed us with indecent, ever larger amounts of chemical preservatives. In the 60's Americans consumed about three pounds of these noxious chemicals, in the 70s about six pounds, and now in the 90s we are reaching the ten pound mark.

Curiously, health officials are not alarmed by the increase in morbidity and mortality caused by fast and convenient unfoods, but morticians are terrified to find corpses, that long ago should have been converted to ashes, fresh as an iceberg lettuce! They report that the average time for a cadaver to decompose now a days is twice as long as 30 years ago. What a trade. The food preservatives accelerate the trip to our graves with the macabre advantage of keeping us presentable longer in our tombs! If only the Pharaohs knew then what we know now.

Because of all the manipulation, modern foods provide us with ridiculously minuscule quantities of nutrients but, thanks to the proactivity of some *health nuts*, there is a growing demand for organically grown produce (fruits and vegetables that are not laden with chemical, pesticides or preservatives). Maureen Kennedy Salaman, a Ph.D. in Nutrition, health activist and author of several books on nutrition said in a conference that nutrients abound in organic vegetables. "A tomato grown by the industry has 2 mg. of magnesium while the organically grown tomato has 2000 mg! The importance of this is paramount since a study in Sidney, Australia, showed a 50% reduction in mortality from cardiovascular diseases when megadoses of magnesium were administered to the patients," she reported.

Why is organic food so nutrient rich? We can only conclude that God has perfectly calculated the loss of nutrients from foods in harvesting, storage and preparation, and has accordingly designed a sufficient quantity of nutrients to be naturally present in them. Yet, as we reject natural laws and take shortcuts, we break this perfect balance and suffer the consequences.

Animals Products

It has been said by experts that a creature who has canine teeth is designed to eat meat. I have no desire to get into trouble with vegetarians, but most of us believe this to be true. Unfortunately, we eat meat as if our canine teeth were a yard long! To supply the enormous demand, the industry has developed scientific methods to increase the production of red and white meats.

For decades health authorities have told us that we need to consume all the protein we can to supply our bodies needs. No sacrifice was too great to bring meat to our tables. Meat producers responded to the challenge with flying colors. In 1940, more than 4 lb. of feed were needed to produce one pound of meat, now in the 90s only 1 lb. is necessary. Another group of foods, dairy products, have been promoted by dietitians and nutritionists as vital. Everybody needs milk, right? Fifty years ago, a cow produced 2,000 pounds of milk per year. Presently, the average milk producers get 50,000 pounds per year per cow. Now, that's what I call efficiency! In my opinion, meat and milk production represent one of the marvels of applied technology. Chemically enhanced feeds, genetic engineering, drugs and hormones are some of the tools used by the modern livestock industry to create the super chickens and monster cows. Dr. Frankenstein's cry, "IT'S ALIVE!" would have been continuous had he this frightening technology.

Consumers now have the information about what they are ingesting, thanks to recent FDA labeling regulations. Unfortunately, most only read the calories and cholesterol amounts. Yet why should we worry? Are not the officials looking after us? In spite of strong complaints, the livestock producers have had preferential treatment; they do not have to list the ingredients of their products. You may think that milk is milk, but the FDA allows the administration of up to 82 drugs to cows in the production of dairy products. Of course, according to the industry, they are beneficial. Bovine growth hormone and estrogen are the most abused; their synergistic effect provokes problems like arthritis, obesity, glucose intolerance, diabetes, heart disease and other less serious but annoying conditions like headaches, fatigue, vision impairment, dizziness, menstrual problems and loss of sexual drive. Of all the drugs used to fatten livestock and tenderize their meat, the most harmful to humans are the female hormones, estrogen. Men are especially worried because they hit us where it hurts the most.

Estrogen

Our world is unnaturally swarming with estrogen and estrogen-like substances. As I mentioned previously, just about all of our foods contain pesticides, most of which have the chemical structure of estrogen and, when ingested, provoke a weak estrogenic effect on our systems. Other estrogen impostors come from the petrochemical industry in the form of plastics used for baby bottles and other plastic recipients. Because of their "weakness" they are considered safe. The problem is the synergism that takes place when combined. The negative effects to our organisms can be devastating.

Inadvertently the livestock feed of a farm in Michigan was contaminated with the pesticide Polychlorinated Biphenyl (PCB), a "weak" estrogen imitator. Pregnant women and mothers that breast fed their children had who consumed the meat of these animals were horrified to find that their male children developed genital deformities and very small penises. In Taiwan, Chinese scientists have under observation 118 male children of mothers that were contaminated with PBC in an accidental spill in 1989. These boys are suffering from the same painful complications as those from Michigan. In lakes with high concentrations of DDT and DDE, pesticides that also have estrogenic effects, the fauna has been severely degenerated. Alligators of the Apopka Lake in Florida have lost virility because of low testosterone and sperm count; consequently the size of their male organs are a fourth of the norm. The Great Lakes are gravely polluted with PCB and DDT. Many fish and seagulls that eat them, have developed grotesque hormonal dysfunction that makes them hermaphrodites, according to Theo Colburn of the Worl d Wildlife Fund.

Niels Skakkebaek, a Danish endocrinologist and probably the foremost authority on the subject of estrogen, reported in 1991 that because of the exaggerated exposure to estrogen and estrogen-like substances, men have presently only 50% of the normal sperm count, significant reduction in the size of their reproductive organs and three times the incidence of testicular cancer. Unbelievable, but John Lennon announced it 30 years ago in his song *Yesterday*: "...Suddenly, I'm just half the man I used to be..." These chemicals have mercilessly maimed our virility, sex drive, fatherhood and manhood. Wives and mothers, if you want more from your husbands, don't feed them estrogen infested meats and foods! Protect your boys (and girls) in the same way.

One could conclude that all this overflow of estrogen was concocted by the women's movement to abolish the "macho" in all men, unfortunately the female hormone also has deteriorated their well-being as well and as bad!

Synthetic estrogens and chemical agents that copy their actions represent a very real threat to society. They are very resistant to breakdown and remain active for a great many years. In one way or another, they end up in the food chain and our body can't neutralize them. Long Island, NY, has the highest incidence of cancer of the breast in the US. Researchers of the NCI have associated it to the vast quantity of pesticides used on the farming soils before they turned to urban communities; now the pesticides are abundant in the local tap water. Mary Wolf, MD, a professor at Mt. Sinai School of Medicine in New York, reported that breast tumor biopsies of women from Long Island showed unusually high concentrations of DDT and DDE. The incidence of cancer was four times higher than in biopsies where the pesticides are absent or in low concentrations.

If the consequences of the "imitators" are this fearful, imagine what the real estrogen found in meats and prescription drugs can do. In spite of the controversy, the research overwhelmingly supports that estrogen increases the incidence of many female ailments including cancer of the breast, uterus and ovaries, among other.

My heart goes out to women. As if the ocean of estrogen that engulfs us was not enough, they have to worry about their own! Their femininity can work against them. The amplitude of their "estrogen window" (lapse between menarche [the first menstruation] and menopause [the last menstruation]) is directly related to the incidence of breast cancer. In other words, if a girl starts her period very young (9 or 10 yr.) and menstruates well into her 50's, she will have greater contact with her endogenous estrogen (produced by herself) and will have higher possibilities of developing this terrible cancer.

Did God make a mistake? The American Cancer Society estimated 11, 000 new cases of breast cancer in 1986. In only a decade, the number rose to 184, 300 for 1996! God is not to blame. The Japanese that eat unsophisticated, low fat, rudimentary diets as well as the Chinese and women from other underdeveloped countries, have extremely low incidence of this type of malignancy. I will explain why further ahead.

But cancer is only one of the many ailments that estrogens have brought upon women. Menstrual, fertility, ovarian and uterine problems can be listed. German scientists have encountered high blood concentrations of PCB in women with endometriosis, an inflammatory pelvic disease that causes severe pre- and menstrual pain, with sterility as one of its major complications. Before the pesticide era, endometriosis was virtually nonexistent. In 1920 only 21 cases had been reported in the whole world. At least five million women presently have endometriosis in the USA alone!

Other Goodies

Again, protection of the product overides the well-being of the consumer. Microorganisms are also the meat grower and dairyman's nightmare. Excessive use of antibiotics both for preventing and treating animal infections, has become an efficient and profitable measure for the food industry and, why not say it, for the drug companies as well. Half of the antibiotics produced are presently consumed by this branch of the food industry. Yet, the antibiotics we ingest in the foods we eat have important deleterious effects. Destruction of friendly bacteria in the throat, colon and vagina give way to fungal infections like candidiasis, a wide spread problem today. Because of our constant inadvertent and involuntary consumption of antibiotics in meat and milk, as well as the ones prescribed, new and resistant strands of bacteria are developing. Pharmacologists have to develop stronger, more expensive and more toxic antibiotics.

Meat packing, like the packing of other products, plays an important role in the livestock industry. Nitrites are another pillar of this industry. They not only preserve meat longer, but give it a cosmetic appeal by intensifying the red color. I already mentioned that when heated, nitrites become carcinogenic. Saliva, tobacco, prescription drugs and some foods have the same effect. These nitrites are widely used in lunch meats, hot dogs and bacon. It was recently published that children who eat 12 or more hot dogs a month are 9.5 times more prone to get leukemia. When mothers consume hot dogs during pregnancy, the incidence of brain cancer in their offspring is greatly increased.

All meats and dairy products are laden with chemicals that one way or another are going to end up in our system. To top it all, the only natural and abundant thing about meat and dairy products is fat (60% of it). The combination of fat and toxic chemicals does sound a bit inconvenient, doesn't it? It seriously increases our chances of developing serious problems like obesity, hypertension, cardiovascular diseases, hyperthyroidism, candidiasis and cancer. According to the General Accounting Office, 143 chemical substances have been detected in commercial meats, 42 are carcinogens and 20 can cause birth defects - none are beneficial!

Of course the healthy livestock and dairy industry is going to fight labeling with all its resources, otherwise a white mustache wouldn't be so appealing any more!

Vegetable Oils

Fat, we all agree, is a major health hazard. Scientists and entrepreneurs are racing to develop healthy fake fat (aha!). Most people admit to food craving, especially the ones loaded with fat and sugar. They taste good, right? Our parents offered desserts as a reward for eating the boring bad-tasting vegetables, grains, and cereals (not frosted flakes of course!).

Scientists came up with the term "mouth feel" to describe "...the uniquely slippery sensation that fat gives to our mouth and tongue." Says Lisa Grunwald of Life magazine, "the average American eats about 11 pounds of cookies a year, 23.6 quarts of ice cream and 11.2 pounds of chocolate on their way to consuming 63.6 pounds of fats and oils."

Certainly, the food industry has not overlooked this monster market opportunity. Yet, for several decades, animal fats have been considered so harmful that experts recommended the consumption of vegetable oils instead. They are obtained from grains, seeds and nuts. For centuries vegetable oils have been used around the world for nutritional, medicinal and religious purposes. Through simple compression of the plants or grains you can obtain excellent quality oils, but, because of their enormous amount of nutrients, they can spoil very quickly. Here we go again! The economically sane thing to do is to find ways to develop vegetable oils with a longer shelf lives.

One ingenious method the experts developed is a process called mechanical extraction. In this process pressure mills crush the seeds and then heat the mass to 240 degrees.

Afterward, the unrefined oil is pressed at over 20 tons of pressure per square inch. This removes from the oil all the elements that can spoil. Unfortunately, all the nutritional value is also lost in the process.

Since these mills are expensive, scientists invented a less machine-intensive, more cost effective method: chemical extraction. This process is obviously preferred by the industry. First, seeds are heated to 160 degrees. Next, they are allowed to rest in gasoline, hexane, ethylene, carbon disulfide, tetrachloride or methyl chloride. The solvent is then evaporated (except for 100 particles per million that remain mixed in the oil , after all, a little poison won't kill you). Finally, through a chlorination process, the carotene is removed. The process yields a crystal clear oil, "degreased" and ready for eternal shelf life (maybe there's a short cut to heaven after all!). Heating and chemical oxidation destroy the nutrients present in the oils. Even worse, the fatty acids in the oil are made toxic by the oxidation process.

It's common knowledge that butter and lard are considered great enemies of health. So, the industry searched for an alternative. Now, by means of high pressure and 380 degree temperatures, oil is hydrogenated and solidified. It is then used in margarine or vegetable shortening, the substitutes for butter and lard. Yet, these chemical substances can't be metabolized by our body. Even worse, they block the utilization of essential oils. With all these health "friends," why do we need enemies?

"Love-Handles Anonymous" keeps pushing the industry to develop tasty and abundant non-fattening products. Chemists have responded to the pressure with a calorie-less fat, totally synthetic food (like plastic). Several years ago, certain companies promised to manufacture something to lower fat calories. In the United States, Nabisco launched a product with the texture of fat, "salatrim," for its cookies. The Nutra-Sweet company put imitation ice creams and sherbets on the market but because their texture was not pleasing to the palate, they stopped producing them. A synthetic fat is used in some frozen desserts (Simplesse), as well as in some cheeses and mayonnaise. And now the FDA has allowed Procter & Gamble a trial with their fake fat Olestra. "Olestra is the stealth missile of fat molecules; it passes through the gastrointestinal tract without being digested or absorbed. As far as the human body is concerned, olestra is fat-free fat," reported Michael D. Lemonick of *Time* magazine. Didn't doctors tell us in the 50's that cigarette smoking was harmless? Scientists, that margarine was better than butter? Common sense dictates that anything fake is, well … fake! These products are damaging to us and the environment.

Refined Products

Sugar

Refined sugar, refined flour, and processed oils are the clearest examples of manufactured foods. They are the core products in the food industry. All other products are envious of their shelf life. They cost almost nothing to produce, and because they are indispensable ingredients in all processed foods, their demand and profitability are scandalous. In fact, the crowning achievement in the food industry was the discovery, 200 years ago, that it was possible to "purify" sugar of any element that might decompose without taking away its sweetness. This process was called "refining."

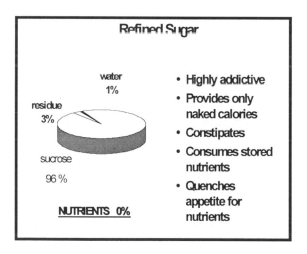

Since its invention in 1751, refined sugar has been the most consumed product worldwide. However, the refining process strips the sugarcane of all its nutritional value. Refined sugar is the prototype of foods without nutritional density. It is composed of 96% sucrose, 3% waste, 1% water and zero nutrients. In other words, its calories are stripped of nutrients, leaving. Another example of "naked calories" is corn syrup. Also known as "anti-nutrients" because on top of not providing nutrients, in order for our organism to utilize them it needs thiamin, riboflavin and niacin, which it draws from the already insufficiently stored nutrients. Coffee, tea and sweets contain mostly naked calories. Since simple carbohydrates require a minimum of work on the part of the organism for their utilization, sugar is rapidly directed to the brain and heart, giving these organs an immediate feeling of energy and well-being and provoking a dependency as strong as any other addictive drug. The restriction of sugar intake produces symptoms typical of withdrawal. Products like these are, alarmingly, the financial backbone of the food industry.

We begin to consume refined sugar almost from birth. Dr. Solarsano, Professor of the University of Guadalajara, Mexico in his article entitled "Collateral Effects of Excessive Consumption of Refined Sugar," reports that sugar is "dangerous for babies and small children." Although many eruptions, infections, allergic reactions and problems of the nervous system disappear when sugar is withdrawn from a child's diet, children are going to demand it because it's highly addictive and destroys the appetite for nutritive foods. Sugar alters the metabolism of calcium and promotes tooth decay. A diet that consists mainly of sugar can bring on many illnesses, including neurosis, hypoglycemia, diabetes mellitus, cancer of the biliary tract, colorectal cancer, arthritis, arteriosclerosis, coronary insufficiency and others.

Public awareness has had a positive impact and the consumption of sugar is rapidly declining. In response to it, the industry has increased the utilization of refined sugar in all processed foods (even salty foods) by 100%. Refined sugar is ubiquitous, involuntarily we are still consuming immoderate amounts. The average American consumes 130 lb. a year and a whopping 66% comes from camouflaged sugar in processed un-foods! Even with the improvement, sugar still constitutes 25% of all the calories the average person ingests.

People who eat less than 30 lb. of sugar per year have a lower incidence of illness and live longer. The Seventh Day Adventists, for example, eat a vegetarian diet and they avoid preservatives and refined foods. It is no coincidence that they live an average of 12 years longer than the rest of the population. There is a direct relationship between the explosion of chronic diseases in the 1940s and the industrialization of sugar in the 1920s. It is the opinion of many that, our problems began when stones mills were replaced by grinders made of iron in the 20s. Incidentally, cereals like wheat and ryes also began to be milled with steel wheels at that time. This, added to the ingesting of processed and canned foods, contributed to an increase in vascular diseases like heart attacks, digestive diseases like diabetes and metabolic diseases like cancer.

Wheat

For many generations, wheat has been the basis of alimentation in many cultures. It is one of the main sources of protein, amino-acids, complex carbohydrates and fiber. Approximately 360 million metric tons of wheat are harvested worldwide each year. We don't get all the benefits we might from wheat because most of it will be or is "refined."

In the process of refining, wheat loses about 80% of vitamin B1 (thiamin), B2 (riboflavin), B3 (niacin) and B6; 98% of vitamin E; 90% of minerals and micronutrients; 80% of biotin; 76% of vitamin K; 75% folic acid; 50% of linoleic acid; 99% of its fiber and it loses about 27 other nutrients. Sorry, I almost forgot to mention the beneficial effect of wheat refinement, it increases its caloric value by 7% (who needs more calories!). Virtual extermination of fiber is the greatest sin of refinement. Let me expound on the forgotten subject of the benefits of fiber and the consequences of its absence. To call the devastation of God designed food a "refinement," is truly blasphemos.

Our health depends on our capacity to nourish ourselves and eliminate waste, everything else is in between. Fiber has the life preserving task of helping our bodies eliminate waste. The result of a fiber poor diet is a chronically constipated society. This condition has perpetuated itself so that even in medical schools they teach us that moving our bowels between once a day and once every three days is normal. Obviously this function is not a priority.

There is no secret that there are ethnic groups who rarely experience disease and who boast impressive life expectancy. From the Himalayans to tribes in Central and South America. Although their eating habits are very different, all live a long time and are seldom ill. What's their secret?

Research groups like H.S. Goldsmith (*Lancet*, 1975) and Reddy and Wynder (*Journal of the National Health Institutes*, 1975) reported that Westerners produce small amounts of feces every 24 to 48 hours, and that their stools are hard, segmented, frequently painful and difficult to excrete. On the other hand, eaters of primitive diets eliminate three times as much waste with soft and voluminous feces that are easy to excrete. Westerners defecate the remains of food eaten two days earlier, while groups like the Hunza report a maximum intestinal transit time of ten hours. The danger of constipation is highly underestimated.

British experts like J. Yuddkin from London in 1972 and later in 1974, T. L. Clave from Bristol, reported high incidence of cancer in peoples from the modern Western world because of diets rich in fats and refined foods. Later Wilkins and Hackman published in (*Cancer Research*, 1974) similar findings in Americans. Their feces contained elevated quantities of nitrogen, fat, cholesterol, biliary acids, and a high concentration of carcinogenic metabolites. Renowned epidemiologist Martin Lipkin published in *Cancer* magazine that groups of Africans, South Americans and Japanese, living in rural areas who eat primitive diets consisting of mainly vegetables, fruits and grains rich in fiber and seldom animal products, have almost no risk of ever developing cancer. These claims are corroborated by the reports of Kian Liu (*Lancet*, 1979) and E. L. Wynder (*Cancer*, 1979) who indicated that for every 100,000 inhabitants in the United States 109 die of colon cancer, but only 4 per every 100,000 in Uganda. This is the quantitative difference between the modern hi-tech diet and a fiber-rich diet.

Dr. Adlercreutz, in his article "Diet, Mammary Cancer and Metabolism of the Sex Hormone," emphasizes that western women enjoy unrestrained consumption of animal proteins and fats, along with refined constipating carbohydrates. This diet not only increases their risk of colon cancer, it substantially increases the production of estrogens. This excessive endogenous estrogen, that normally should be eliminated through the stool, is trapped in the colon because of constipation and is easily reabsorbed back into the already unnaturally excessive bloodstream concentration. In contrast, Oriental women and others that adhere to natural unadulterated foods, avoid this deadly vicious cycle because their diets are low in fats, animal protein and refined products. They consume foods high in fiber like fruits, vegetables and grains. Thanks to proper, easy, frequent evacuations, their exposure to hormones is closer to the ideal because of no excess production due to poor diet and no recycling.

But not all estrogens are harmful. There are estrogens both good and bad. The most abundant is 16-hydroxyesterone which damages DNA causing among other problems, mammary and testicular cancer. The most common of the good ones is 2-hydroxyesterone which even has cancer preventing properties. Vegetables such as the soybean, broccoli and the pomegranate, offer us phyto-hormones or phyto-estrogens which protect us from carcinogenic mutations. Chinese and Japanese women not only are less exposed to the excess of endogenous estrogens, they also consume foods rich in good estrogen like tofu, soy and miso, a thick fermented paste made by grinding together cooked soybeans, rice or barley. Consequently their first menstruation comes in their late teens, menopause in their mid- forties and they never have hormone replacement therapy because they consume foods with "good" phyto-hormones. As a result, they seldom develop cancer and, curiously, they rarely suffer osteoporosis or any of the diseases related to low endogenous estrogen production of menopause. Even though there are many contrasts in the primitive diets around the world, the common denominator is the abundance of nutritious natural foods and fiber.

Other Consequences of Ingesting Processed Foods

Our overfed-undernourished-disease-prone scientists "think" that enriching the processed un-foods with a few synthetic vitamins is going to make up for their mischievous technological manipulations. If you think that their minds have not been affected by malnutrition, think again!

Lack of nutritious meals and pollution have gravely affected our IQs. Unfortunately, it doesn't stop there. According to multiple university investigations, the serious increase in behavioral problems in children and adolescents is directly connected to diet and poor nutrition. The present day diet of adolescents consists mainly of junk food. Pathological aggressiveness in children and teenagers is related to the consumption of the refined sugars found in sweets and sodas. Jails are a showcase for this behavioral problem. In one of them a dietary experiment was carried out where sweets, cookies, and sodas were exchanged for fruit, fresh vegetables, and water. Aggressiveness and other behavior problems among the prisoners diminished remarkably in just a couple of weeks! This simple, inexpensive experiment clearly demonstrates the relationship between behavioral problems and diet.

Vitamin and mineral deficiencies affect the biochemical balance which controls the neurotransmitters in the brain, according to researchers from the Massachusetts Institute of Technology. This crucial alteration leads to learning and behavioral dysfunction. It took them a while to make this discovery, considering that in 1790 (not 1970!) at the Tuke's Clinic in York, England, complete wards of patients diagnosed with dementia were emptied when a regiment of nutritious foods was implemented.

In the Cleveland Clinic, a group of 20 teenagers with neurotic problems were found to have a severe thiamin deficiency. After failure to treatment with conventional methods, the doctors treated them with thiamin instead. The alternative (often disapproved) treatment produced either marked improvement or total remission of the symptoms. Thiamin, also called vitamin B1, is necessary for carbohydrate metabolism and normal neural activity. Lack of thiamin causes beriberi, a disease which can cause neurological symptoms, behavioral dysfunction, disorientation and delirium. Vitamin B3 deficiency also causes Pellagra, a disease characterized by psychiatric symptoms such as dementia as well as depression, diarrhea and skin problems.

Oftentimes, children with attention deficit disorders and hyperactivity are prescribed dangerous drugs like Ritalin. Many times these symptoms are caused from a deficiency in "B" vitamins (beriberi, pellagra) due to high consumption of refined sugar and flour that mimics the already poor deposits of thiamin. Nothing a good diet can't resolve -provide children with natural unadulterated produce, restrict refined sugar and flours and give them a good helping of thiamin.

Drug addiction is probably the worst symptom of decay in our society. If we would concentrate more efforts into changing our eating habits, our children would have more resources to avoid drugs. At Oasis Hospital in Tijuana, Mexico, we treated 100 youngsters with chronic addiction to heroin or cocaine who had failed to respond to other conventional treatments.

Our treatment consisted of intensive intravenous infusions of vitamins, minerals, amino acids, and a complete change in their eating habits. All of them left the hospital drug free after 15 days. After one year, the follow up report indicated that 60% were still sober. Of course spiritual and emotional support is vital, but when you compare the results from the literature of conventional management of addictions at 17%, it is ridiculous that proper nutrition is overlooked.

All this research and money has been spent to prove the obvious! Yet, despite all these logical findings, health authorities, medical doctors and other health professionals are not taking advantage of the benefits that nutrition can bring in reducing the incidence and mortality of many diseases. The thing that really amazes me is that doctors do not recognize any relationship between diet and brain function (behavior, learning capacity, etc.), proof enough that they are eating too much junk! Their only "brain food" is reading medical journals which, as I will expose, has resulted in atrocious judgmental errors.

Taking into account that the consumption of technologically manipulated foods is a major cause of cardiovascular diseases, cancer and many other illnesses, I have to agree with those who say that more people have died from consuming refined food products than have died in all the wars combined. Even though research abounds on the subject, inexcusably the food industry continues to envenom society, and doctors just watch. I guess that's the profitable thing to do. How could they attack the industry that provides most of their clientele? Furthermore, I question the integrity of the services the medical industry provides to the "clientele."

Chapter 4

111:
The Doctor's
Number

> But their understanding was futile and their foolish hearts
> weredarkened. Professing themselves to be
> wise they became fools.

The Apostle Paul

Sickness is a natural consequence of living surrounded by adversaries that attack us from within and from without. Not to worry, our lives are safe because of unprecedented advances in medical science, new knowledge and amazing technology is at our service to counteract the ravages of our world. But, how safe are we really?

A Select Group

In 1978, after taking the medical board exams, a group of my fellow graduates and I asked some of our professors what specialties we should pursue. One of my colleagues was interested in infectology. Our professors were of the opinion that infectology would be an extinct specialty because scientific advances in pharmacology were so promising that surely there would soon be antibiotics to eradicate every kind of infection. I felt proud and at the same time unworthy to be part of a group of scientists that could have such an impact on the future of humanity. While my comrades deliberated the specialty they would enter, I was set on surgery. I had made that decision many years earlier when I accepted that my future as a pianist was limited. I also considered becoming a cartoonist but I couldn't even write my name legibly. It was apparent by my poor penmanship that I was destined to be a doctor. So, at age 14, I decided to become a surgeon. No other branch of medicine was of interest to me.

When I finished my studies at the University of the State of Mexico, I possessed all the enthusiasm and innocence of a typical graduate. After being accepted to the University Hospital in Vienna, Austria, the cradle of surgery, I began my residency in oncological surgery with a scholarship from the Mexican government.   It was more than an honor to be in an institution with eight Nobel Prizes to its credit and home to Theodor Billroth, Hans Finsterer and Karl Landsteiner. These doctors are to surgeons what Bill Gates is to computer enthusiasts. The University of Vienna is also the alma mater of Sigmund Freud and many other physicians that have made it into the history books. I was so thrilled to be there that I never objected to the long shifts. At times I would spend up to 72 hours straight in the operating room with a seemingly endless stream of patients. I suffered varying degrees of sleep deprivation during those five years, but it was worth it. I was becoming what I had wanted to be for so long. Not only was I learning surgical techniques from the best, but they shared with me a deeply conservative criteria. A criteria that was patient-centered. Diseased centered criteria, not by the all powerful medical institutions of America, prevails in most parts of the world. I feel blessed that I attended a school where the professors focused on the patient, not the disease.

As I finished my specialty and left the safety of the university environment, still enthusiastic and innocent, I decided to avoid the cold and mechanized "real" world of modern science. I wanted to help the sick with good old-fashioned medicine. But to ignore the medical "new order" mandated by American institutions is to commit professional suicide. The United States is the leader in the modernization and mechanization of medicine. No one has invested more time, effort, and money in the development of awesome technology such as Computerized Tomography Scans, Magnetic Resonance Imagers, lasers, video surgery components, etc. These costly "toys" fascinate doctors everywhere the way Super Nintendo has captured the attention of our children. Though the rest of the world loves to criticize the Americans for the automation of medicine, they are desperately trying to emulate them. Even the University of Austria is giving in to the temptation because medical technology has a spell-casting attraction so powerful that we, the doctors, are as dependent on it as addicts are to their drugs.

The achievement that must truly be credited to the American medical industry is the creation of an omnipotent medical marketing machine. It has completely convinced doctors everywhere that America has divine knowledge and that all should strive to be like its doctors. The super technology and super specialties make a doctor feel like Superman. As a result, surgeons act faster than a speeding bullet to get more patients on the operating table. Yes, the medical establishment is stronger than a locomotive but I fear that its patients are tied down to the train tracks. It is easy to run over your patients once you have dehumanized them by forgetting about the person and focusing only on the disease. Today's doctors are able to leap over a patient's feelings in a single bound.

The reading of the Hippocratic Oath still brings tears to the eyes of many doctors. I believe that there still exists altruistic humans behind the cold stethoscopes. However, the pressure to keep up with the overwhelming medical information, the costs of malpractice insurance, the stress of dealing with the sick and the dying (especially when according to the establishment, there are no answers to many diseases like cancer) makes it easier to detach yourself from patients. I'm reminded of that old adage used to admonish the servant of God: "Don't get so wrapped up doing the work of God that you forget the God of the work." Doctors are so preoccupied with the disease of the patient that they forget about the patient who has the disease. Hippocrates, the father of medicine, would tell those doctors that the patient comes first. Always.

The Medical Industry

In the following pages, I will express my very personal opinion about the status of the practice of modern medicine based on my 20 years of experience, and that of other authors who have dedicated themselves to the evaluation of the medical industry.

Although the "medical industry" encompasses a wide variety of businesses, agencies and services, I will dedicate this chapter to the main providers: doctors, pharmaceutical laboratories, and hospitals.

Achievements in the Field of Medicine

The second half of this century has seen the greatest technological explosion in the history of medicine - chemical syn-
theses of pharmaceuticals, genetic engineering, computeriza-
tion in microbiology, nuclear medicine, gamma knife, trans-
plants, endoscopic surgery, surgical training simulators, and
hundreds of other scientific advances. In the clinical field,
new devices facilitate the work of physicians. Computer programs exist which diagnose and recommend a treatment. It is
now possible to examine organs using a tiny probe that functions as a video camera. New technology permits accident
victims to be attended to rapidly by teams of highly trained
doctors, nurses, and technicians, that often bring patients
"back" to life. In our Hospital, The Oasis of Hope, in Tijuana,
Mexico we have living proof of the benefits of these advances.
Francisco Bucio M.D., one of our plastic surgeons, was a victim of the devastating earthquake in Mexico City in 1985. At
the time he was working in a hospital that collapsed while he
was making his rounds. When they rescued him, 4 fingers
from his right hand had been so destroyed they had to be amputated and only the thumb could be saved. He thought his
career had ended but a fellow plastic surgeon from the US
transposed two toes, the longest from each foot, to his damaged hand. He now has opposing "fingers" to the thumb and a
functional hand. Isn't it unbelievable? Wait, there's more, he
also is one of the busiest plastic surgeons in our city due to
his excellent abilities.

Now, that's what I call a miracle! Then why am I so critical about modernization and technology? It's because I'm disillusioned about the achievements (or lack of) in the ailments that most affect our population Yes, medicine has come a long way. But we are in awe and can't take our eyes and minds off the glitter of the machinery, while losing sight of the patient.

These technological creations undeniably represent a huge advance in the diagnosis and treatment of diseases but no apparatus or computer program can replace the human touch of a doctor. The abuse of technology has undermined the ability of the physician to listen to and observe the patient. Modernization saves doctors time and effort, unfortunately we are allocating this saved time to the development of more and more devices instead of taking advantage of it to dedicate more attention to patients, especially those with chronic diseases that need a lot of our time. On the contrary, consultation times are increasingly shorter and doctors distance themselves more from patients. The lure of technology has alienated physicians from their mission.

It seems to me that these days we spend all our time learning how to use the new gadgets that are substituting the obsolete ones that only arrived last month! My father, Ernesto Contreras Sr., MD, a doctor from the old school of medicine, instilled in me a philosophy that is not opposed to progress but disagrees with anything that places the patient as a secondary concern.

The original mission of medicine was established some 500 years before Christ. It was shaped into the following oath, a pact physicians make with society. One version, approved by the American Medical Association, is as follows:

You do solemnly swear, each by whatever he or she holds most sacred

That you will be loyal to the Profession of Medicine and just and generous to its members

That you will lead your lives and practice your art in uprightness and honor

That into whatsoever house you shall enter, it shall be for the good of the sick to the utmost of your power, your holding yourselves far aloof from wrong, from corruption, from the tempting of others to vice

That you will exercise your art solely for the cure of your patients, and will give no drug, perform no operation, *for a criminal purpose*, even if solicited, far less suggest it

That whatsoever you shall see or hear of the lives of men or women which is not fitting to be spoken, you will keep inviolably secret

These things do you swear. Let each bow the head in sign of acquiescence

And now, if you will be true to this, your oath, *may prosperity and good repute be ever yours*; the opposite, if you shall prove yourselves forsworn.

The Hippocratic Oath

As we will see, we have departed far from this philosophy, from the commitment that all doctors have made to society! Conveniently, some changes were made from the original oath. It called for doctors not to provoke abortions and lastly, the penalty for not complying even in part, was death. In Mexico we say that fear doesn't walk like a donkey. Americans would say that fear is quicker than lightning.

I strongly believe that the forefathers of modern medicine did heroic deeds, but they were under tremendous, understandable, pressure, as I will explain, that took us down the wrong path. Let's review my critical, negative analysis from a historical point of view.

Epidemics and the Birth of The Medical Industry

Epidemics have killed a vast number of people. Jean Hamburger, a French researcher, in his book *Honey and Hemlock*, exposes the tragedy of these deaths. The impression left in those that experienced the raging fury of death during that period can easily be perceived reading his words:

"I have seen the wounded stare of too many men, women, young people and children even who foresaw themselves as damned because they could not understand that whole races of people had made the diseases a sign of the wrath of the gods."

The black plague killed 25 million Europeans in the 1300s, cholera claimed the lives of 100,000 Frenchman in 1832, typhus claimed 3 million Poles and Russians in 1914, and again in Europe, the flu epidemic killed 25 million people in 1918.

We can't begin to imagine what the people laid low by these epidemics suffered. Perhaps we can get a vague idea of what the Europeans suffered when we see news about the horror of cholera or ebola. Although it is true that cancer, cardio-vascular diseases, and AIDS affect hundreds of thousands of people around the world, they can't be compared to the epidemics of the past. In the late Middle Ages, the common epidemics were malaria, leprosy, typhus, influenza and St. Anthony's Fire. Perhaps the pestilence that desolated Europe the most was The Black Death, a bubonic plague of the pulmonary type. The Black Death began around 1333 in the central region of Asia, later extending itself to the Mediterranean Sea, Russia and Ireland, reaching its climax in 1348. It is said that one-fourth of the population died in places stricken by it. Physicians considered isolation as the only recourse. So it was that the "quarantine" was born near the end of the 15th century.

At the end of the 15th century, syphilis took on epidemic characteristics, not respecting social class, rank or sex. The name of the disease follows a legend about a young shepherd called Syphilo who had this disease imposed on him for insulting the Sun. It spread rapidly among his companions. It is said that the Renaissance was lashed by two plagues, syphilis and witch hunts. The latter was converted into a true collective psychosis. The witches were nothing more than women with mental dysfunction who, since not recognized as ill, fell under the jurisdiction of the theologians and lawyers instead of the care of a physician. They are also known from the Salem (Massachusetts) trials of the 17th century when a series of women were executed for witchcraft. We know now that their actions and behavior were caused by foods containing spores of hallucinogenic mushrooms with alkaloids similar to LSD. Thanks to 20 years of research, Dr. Johannes Weyer in his book *Diabolical Frauds* along with contemporary scientific discoveries, the hereditary stain has been removed from many families who believed they had witches in their ancestry.

In the 17th century, some new diseases were identified: rickets, tuberculosis and beriberi. Smallpox attacked Europe in the 18th century but an important medical event contributed to the fight against it —immunization, a method based on the principle that people who survive a forced attack are protected from future attacks. Therefore, if a person was exposed to a light attack, he was protected from the epidemic. In that century, Edward Jenner appeared on the scene. He was a rural British doctor who found out about this folk belief that people who contracted "cowpox" would not contract smallpox. Jenner made the belief the subject of experimentation for two years and in 1796 injected into a child purulent secretions of cowpox. Six weeks later, he injected the subject with the pus of smallpox. He observed absolutely no symptom of smallpox in the child. So it was that a new therapy was born. Since it was obtained from cattle (vacca in Latin) it was called a vaccination.

Before the advent of these scientific advances, the authorities used desperate methods to try and control epidemics. They buried corpses together with all their belongings and burned them; in some cases even entire cities. They petitioned the heavens and offered all sorts of sacrifices. Some placed the blame on Jews and in desperation and hatred, massacred 600 in Brussels and 2000 in Strasbourg.

Up to this time, scientists could do nothing but just stand as spectators of the plague's hurricanes. But the invention of the microscope and the discovery of the germ brought light on the cause of these devastating infectious plagues. For the first time, doctors were able to look their enemies in the face. Death did not come as a result of chance, divine providence, the Jews or the wrath of God!

With the enemy in sight, the fear of God was extrapolated to the fear of germs. So doctors, immunologists, microbiologists, physiologists and many other specialists began to wage war against an infinitely smaller but tremendously resourceful foe. Their scientific drive, restricted for so many centuries, emerged with a passionate force that could not be stopped. There was excitement and hope for the physician; hope of achieving the victory over infectious diseases caused by these insolent, minuscule microbes.

Doctors and Health

In this scientific environment of the mid 19th century, two opposing schools of thought were born, headed by two gigantic figures, Bernard and Pasteur. In the matter of the development of disease, what was black for one was white for the other.

Claude Bernard (1813-1870), French physician and physiologist, was the first to consider that the body's ability to mend depends on its general condition, that is to say, how nourished it is. If our body can depend on an adequate internal environment, Bernard asserted that it will know how to make the necessary adjustments to maintain the proper state of balance. He concluded that germs are only responsible for the development of disease if our body offers conditions favorable to the germ. If our body maintains an adequate *"milieu intérieur"* or internal environment, it will be able to fight off the germ and there will be no disease. It seemed like an irrefutable argument. How else could one explain the fact that, though we all come in contact with the same germs, only a few of us fall ill? This is the fundamental theory of the **humorist** school of thought. Of course Bernard was a man with a sense of humor, but the purpose of calling the movement "humorist" was to give honor to Hippocrates who 500 years before Christ, without the help of microscopes, knew that there were "forces within us that truly heal." The ancient Greeks believed that the body was formed by four "humors" (Latin for liquids). Any alteration in their perfect balance caused pain, disease, even emotional changes; hence the modern application of saying "good or bad humor."

Louis Pasteur (1822-1895), on the other hand, disagreed with Bernard, affirming that germs are the true villains in the history of disease and that by neutralizing them, we not only could prevent infections, we could also cure them. His hypothesis was confirmed by his vaccines and treatments. This is the fundamental theory of the **causalist** school of thought, so named because if the **cause** of a disease can be determined, the saving antidote can be developed.

Pasteur's prestige is founded on his accomplishments in microbiology. The research and experiments he conducted led to the confirmation of his hypothesis in 1877. Pasteur demonstrated that germs reproduce themselves like any other organism.These advances formed the guiding principles of disease control research. Today, many owe their life to the achievements of Pasteur, but the methods employed in his research were reckless.

One of his achievements is the vaccine against rabies, but with no more clinical data than that of Jenner, he prepared the vaccine, gave it to a healthy volunteer (fool) and then infected him with the disease! Pasteur and his colleagues must have had many anxious hours and days waiting for the deadly outcome, but the "guinea pig" survived and was declared successfully inoculated. This experiment got everybody's attention and gave him even more notoriety than before, in the eyes of scientists and the public. Soberly and humbly, the genius he was, said, "Luck favors the prepared minds." Pasteur frequently departed from the scientific method established in his day and carried out experiments that were neither very ethical nor humane.

One of the great misfortunes of being human is the fact that we spend so much time waiting. What we want is action and quick results. Because of this, when Pasteur opened the door to the search for the illusive germ and provided the weaponry for the fight, the world, scientific and not, was ready to take the initiative. Almost everyone followed Pasteur and the causalist school of thought, of course! The French government responded and funded a research institute for Pasteur to continue with the exploration of microorganisms, so the Pasteur Institute opened its door in 1886. To date this research institute is at the forefront of scientific discovery; the last one attributed to them was the Human Immundeficiency Virus (HIV).

When I think of Pasteur, as well as other physicians and scientists of the 19th and 20th centuries, I feel like a single brick lying beside the Sears Tower in Chicago, Illinois, because those doctors were models of dedication. They truly laid down their lives for the pure joy of discovery. Think, for example, of Elie Metchnikoff (1845-1916), Russian biologist and pathologist who discovered phagocytes and situated himself in Paris to be able to work with Pasteur and his institute. With the passing of the years, he was able to absorb the "advances" in the struggle against infection but his observations and research obliged him to question the theory of Pasteur. Soon, he switched to Claude Bernard's humorist school of thought. Metchnikoff wanted to show the importance of the humorist's perspective, but few paid attention to his work because Pasteur wasn't in agreement. In order to make his point clear, Metchnikoff and several co-workers stood before an assembly of physicians and drank a liquid contaminated with millions of cholera bacilli. They did this to demonstrate their conviction that if the immune system is strong, it has the power to resist germs. Metchnikoff demonstrated his hypothesis in an overwhelming way. Not a single one of the participants in the experiment fell ill with cholera. Although the course of history was not changed, Metchnikoff gained respect, so much so that Pasteur named him as his successor in 1904.

He continued with his studies in immunology and physiology and won the Nobel price for Medicine in 1908.

In the second half of the 19th century and the first two decades of the 20th, the two most feared germs of all time were discovered. Robert Koch (1843-1910) discovered these germs which cause tuberculosis and cholera and received the Nobel Prize for his work in 1905. Other germs were discovered that cause typhoid fever, gonorrhea, malaria, diphtheria, amoebiasis, tetanus, meningitis, syphilis and rubella. These accomplishments pushed scientists toward a search for treatments that would specifically seek out germs without causing any damage to normal cells. This concept was called "magic bullet" and continues to be the guiding principle of the modern day pharmaceutical industry. The truth is that any medication that enters the body is exposed to thousands of barriers, both physical and chemical, and its success depends on the reaction of each particular person. Some medications can have beneficial effects but they can also be converted into morbid substances and be lethal as we shall observe later.

Paul Ehrlich is considered the father of the pharmaceutical industry. He was the first to produce pharmaceuticals in an organized way. Another highly important event was the accidental discovery of Penicillin in 1928 by Alexander Fleming (1881-1955). Fleming had been engaged in the search for causative agents in the influenza epidemic of 1918 which did away with 25 million people. On a holiday he left

his bacterial cultures on the work table in his London laboratory. They became contaminated with green fungus which destroyed the microorganisms of the culture. There is no doubt
that "luck favors the prepared". This "luck" earned him the
Nobel Prize in 1945.

As a direct result, the massive production of antibiotics began and since then, doctors and researchers have not looked
back; they have devoted themselves to the mission of con-
quering the infectious insolent bugs that cause diseases. The
success of antibiotics guaranteed the causalist's school of
thought to flourish. It has become an immovable and incontrovertible institution. Those who oppose it today are disregarded without a backward glance because the statutes of the
establishment are medical dogma. To belong to it is a privilege, to oppose it is heresy. Its principles and laws are even
protected by a myriad of governmental agencies and societies like the National Health Institutes and the American Cancer Society.

Engineers and Health

The improvement in worldwide health is attributed, by the
medical industry, to the development of drugs that destroy
causal agents. The truth is that the control of plagues and
disease has been achieved because of sociological changes
like hygiene, better distribution of food and, however unre-
lated to health it may seem, city planning. I would almost
dare to affirm that public health problems diminished

in great measure because of these factors long before a vaccination was injected and the first "magic bullet" administered. For example, the appropriate management of sewage in the 18th century and the practice of quarantine yielded impressive results, but the deplorable living conditions of those far away times are for us now inconceivable. Some time ago I read a book by Patrick Sueskind, *The Perfume* that, even though it's a novel, describes with exquisite precision the environment of Paris in the 18th century (if you are eating, I recommend you read this later):

> In the period that interests us reigned stench scarcely conceivable to modern man. The streets reeked of manure, house yards stank of urine, halls and stairways smelled of rotting wood and rat excrement, kitchens were redolent of rotting cabbage and mutton fat, unventilated bedrooms stank of moldy dust, sleeping places smelled of greasy sheets, of humid quilts and the penetrating sweetish odor of urinals. Fireplaces stank of sulfur, canneries of caustic bleaches, slaughter houses of coagulated blood. Men and women stank of sweat and dirty clothing. In their mouths was the pestilence of infected teeth. Their breath smelled of onions and their bodies, when no longer young, of rancid cheese, sour milk and malignant tumors. The river stank, the city square stank, churches reeked and the same stench was breathed under bridges and in palaces. Clergy stank noless than country folk, the craftsman no more than the teacher'swife. The whole of the nobility stank and even the king stank like a

carnivorous beast and the queen like an old goat, winter was no different than summer because in the 18th century they hadn't yet put a stop to the corrosive activity of bacteria and thus there was no human action, creative or destructive, no manifestation of life incipient or in decadence, that was not accompanied by some offensive odor.

If the inhabitants of the most progressive city of Europe lived under such nauseating conditions, the circumstances of the rest of the old world belong to the unthinkable. Obviously in these miserable conditions diseases spread like wild fire, but to science this was not so obvious, especially to medical science. In 1847 Dr. Ignas Semmelweis was ousted from the medical profession for the "quackery" of promulgating that doctors should wash their hands before exploring their patients. At that time they would do an autopsy and, without washing their hands, explore a patient! And these are the guys that supposedly have a better than average IQ, scary!

Let history speak instead. Thanks to improvements in sewage and general sanitation, smallpox epidemics began a dizzying descent before Edward Jenner discovered inoculation. Smallpox might actually have disappeared without any treatment at all. But doctors had to intervene and the general use of vaccination was popularized. Curiously, the incidence of this disease began to ascend at the end of the 19th century. By 1892, the number of people infected with smallpox had ascended to 165,774 more cases than in the years preceding vaccination. In 1865, an alarming increase in death by smallpox was reported in England. More than 22,000 died after vaccination became obligatory there. By 1872, over 44,000 deaths were reported and the number of fatalities continued to climb each year in spite of vaccination. It took officials 76 years to wake up to the fact that the vaccine was the real cause of the deaths.

In 1939, Germany instituted obligatory vaccination against diphtheria and the incidence of this disease rose astronomically to 150,000. Norway, on the other hand, decided not to vaccinate. Only 50 cases were reported there in the same period. Another greatly feared epidemic in the

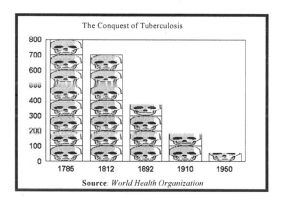

19th century was tuberculosis. In 1812, the death rate from tuberculosis in New York was 700 lives for every 100,000 inhabitants. By 1892, the rate had diminished to 370 and further to 180 in 1910. By 1950, the rate stood at 50 lives per 100,000. The need for the treatment has to be seriously questioned since the downward trend would probably have continued without the treatment. Statistics demonstrate that infant mortality from scarlet fever, diphtheria, whooping cough and mumps diminished 90% between 1869 and 1896, before the introduction of antibiotics and immunization. It shouldn't be surprising that Pasteur, on his deathbed, was quoted as confessing to Metchnikoff, "the pathogen (germ) is nothing, the terrain is everything" referring to the internal environment that Bernard had postulated.

Yet, medical science did not change its trajectory. The search for "magic bullets" that will destroy germs continues. I guess it's the profitable thing to do. In our time, Native Americans have the highest infant mortality, suffer infectious diseases in epidemic proportions and are cursed with the shortest longevity in the nation. Philanthropists decided to resolve the Navajos' health problems by making generous donations to back a program designed by the University of Cornell's Medical School. The program was implemented in 1960.

A full fledged clinic, with all the technological advances of the time, was constructed for the project and highly trained Cornell physicians were sent to attend the Navajo full time. After five years of dedicated and arduous work by all involved, the Cornell-Navajo project was terminated. Medical knowledge, technology and drugs had no impact on infant mortality which continued at 300% higher than the nation's average. Infectious diseases were not put under control and the longevity of Native Americans did not improve. On average, they die 11 years before most Americans. The rate of death by tuberculosis diminished insignificantly and continues to be 11 times higher than the rest of the country.

The living conditions of Native Americans is deplorably similar to 17th century Europeans. Efforts to improve their health should be spent on infrastructure to improve their environment rather than sending in medical brigades.

The power of the medical industry's propaganda is truly omnipotent; it not only has obscured the eyes of the doctors and scientists but also of the rest of the world. Our hearts tell us that we have the power to listen to our body and know what is happening to it. Sadly, scientific criteria have clouded our instincts, convincing us that we were foolish. How else do we explain that it has taken 100 years to realize the causalist school offers only a mirage. How can "the establishment" keep offering us a myth and call it truth?

As I learn more of the medical failures and the absurd measures we partake in order to justify ourselves, the words of the Apostle Paul hit me in the face: "...Professing themselves to be wise, they became fools" (Romans 1:22). I realize that he was not referring to physicians or scientists but, although uncomfortable, it applies well. Wait, it gets worse ... fools with tools are cruel and dangerous!

The Pharmaceutical Industry

Since the beginning of the industrially produced pharmaceuticals, it was obvious that governments needed to establish and maintain some rules of production in order to protect the consumer. The public health departments of many countries require that laboratories comply with all the rules. Pharmaceutical laboratories are assigned registration numbers and licenses to produce, distribute and sell drugs proven to be "safe and effective." These registers, permits, registration numbers or licenses are the most valuable possessions of the pharmaceutical industry. The requirements are always evolving. They have been modified and made more sophisticated, complicated, and ridiculously expensive. Nevertheless, in large measure, they continue to be useless as far as protecting the consumer is concerned.

Throughout the world, governmental authorities "look out" for our interests and our health. The need to control pharmaceuticals from the very start of the manufacturing process is important because they are dangerous. But the ruling powers that determine when and how they will be delivered to the ill are not always aimed toward the well-being of the patient. Ahead of the patients come the investors who keep a watchful eye on the security of their money and astutely measure the probability of success (economic of course). Next come the producers with their scientific equipment who also worry about their share of the profits, and way down the list comes the "well-being" of the patient.

As an example of this, I will mention the first industrially elaborated medicine. Remember that Paul Ehrlich received a Nobel Prize in 1908. Ehrlich developed an effective drug against syphilis, the first compound known as a "magic bullet" **salvarsan**. This treatment was used all over Europe and America by the name Triparsamide. It was produced by Merck Laboratories and backed by the American Medical Association (AMA) who promoted its massive distribution in spite of the fact that Ehrlich had previously recommended its use be abandoned when he discovered that it caused blindness, due to destruction of the optic nerve, in an elevated percentage of patients.

Marketing Opportunities

The pharmaceutical industry, indecently profitable, deals with diseases not as afflictions but as market opportunities. For instance AIDS, the newest market, has had the advantage of rapid growth and less resistance from the FDA to try treatments with some "short cuts" because of the enormous pressure patients and activists are putting on the US government to find a cure. In 1985, the National Institute of Health (NIH) invited Burrows-Welcome, an English company with experience in antivirals (owners of the patent for the popular anti-flu Sudafed) to develop and manufacture a treatment against the devastating plague.

Researchers of the laboratory immersed themselves in the archives of the pharmacological junk yard and came up with a anti-cancer drug (chemotherapy) known for its antiviral activity, AZT, rejected by the FDA 23 years earlier as being primitive and extremely toxic. But the NIH gave in to the "pressure" of the epidemic and began its clinical application. The risk is acceptable since the patients were sentenced to die. Interestingly, close to 600,000 patients are in the same situation every year who are going to die of cancer and any type of alternative is absolutely prohibited! Without losing any time, Burrows-Welcome requested a patent which was granted in 1988. The first study concluded that AZT did not prolong the life of AIDS victims but did improve their quality of life, an interesting conclusion, given the fact that it had been discontinued in the 70s precisely because of severe side effects. Harvard University also carried out clinical testing with AZT on patients in advanced stages of AIDS in which it was noted that this "improvement in their quality of life" consisted of retarding the onset of typical symptoms. The results were counterproductive since the patient suffered more from the side effects of AZT therapy (nausea, vomiting, fatigue, etc.). By 1992, the sales of AZT had topped 100 million dollars, thanks to the sales pitch based on its ephemeral benefits.

As is to be expected, pharmaceutical laboratories -large and small- wanted a "piece of the market" but instead of cooperating and sharing scientific experience, greed divided them. As in all wars, disunity weakened them and none have been able to defeat this minuscule but powerful virus. In the 80s everyone was in a race against time to find a treatment or a vaccine. After barely ten years of arduous research, Merck announced that they would stop participating in the race, owing to the enormous mutation capacity of the virus, its resistance to antivirals, a very doubtful market and a very poor perspective for finding an effective treatment, they were suspending their anti-AIDS program. The pharmaceutical industry, its investors, and scientists forgot about the global consequences that this epidemic could cause and almost all of them abandoned AIDS "research." In other words, they no longer had any interest in this "market."

Responsibility to the Consumer

The case of AZT is just one example of how health departments, here and abroad, do not always protect us from toxic or ineffective pharmaceuticals. They never make or repeat studies on their own. They simply approve or disapprove a drug on the basis of the studies of scientifically established research to which the pharmaceutical industry zealously adheres. Out of all this play acting, what government officials do seek is what happens to the guinea pigs. Effectiveness is measured in terms of desirable overriding undesirable effects; if a few thousand must suffer or die, it's part of science. The pharmaceutical laboratories get rich either way.

Institutional and Professional Ethics

None of the pharmaceutical firms will deny that most research is done "in house." They also have recourse to independent institutions who "impartially" corroborate their findings in order to help them gain the trust of the authorities and the public. Until a short time ago, universities carried out their functions in an unbiased manner. Supposedly they didn't allow themselves to be influenced by the economic incentives, officially called "donations" and "scholarships," offered by the industry. Yet, it is hard to believe that a university or research group would find a drug or product even potentially dangerous and run the risk of losing these subsidies. Recently, David Letterman said that the researchers who found cigarette smoking to be NON-addictive should be nominated for the Nobel Prize! I guess the tobacco industry moguls (not their scientists) are not smoking and are eating healthy brain foods that keep them quite sharp in order to come up with such an incredible scientific scam!

Most universities no longer hide the fact that they are business partners in the development of products and claim a share in patents and earnings. Sumner Slichter of Harvard University expressed it eloquently. "The discovery that an enormous amount of research can be carried on for profit is surely one of the most revolutionary economic discoveries of the century." As we say in Mexico, "off with the masks!"

Knowledge and teaching were the foundations of the great schools but in this present age, their mission has been compromised. They have sold out because of greed. Harvard has given more presidents to the United States that any other university; six in all. It has been granted 33 Nobel Prizes and 25 Pulitzer Prizes. It has formed thousands of authors and generated inventions that have impacted humanity. In the industrial world it is now known as the "central bank of ideas and inventors." Today's Harvard, along with other research institutions, is a profitable business, where its products are science and scientists. The Pasteur Institute is not far behind. They have the record at 254 patents, 75 products under licensing and 360 biological substances protected pending their patent. No wonder they have clones; there are 23 Pasteur Institutes sprinkled throughout the world. The fusion of the biomedical research with money is an enormous ethical contradiction, yet this marriage between science and business has been unashamedly productive. Universities now upgrade their academic level so that their research will have greater commercial value.

In all human activity, from playing marbles to publishing an article about the life threatening effects of a drug, cheating happens. If universities and research institutions were totally independent of the economic influence of the industry, would the results be more honest? The esteem we hold for scientists is often so exalted that it seems like we would put our hands in the fire for them. Their integrity, we think, is as clean as their lab coats. The harsh reality shatters this perception. Gerald Geison, a Historian from the University of Princeton was able to study Pasteur's lab notes, zealously kept by the family over 100 years, and determined that Pasteur's anthrax vaccine was actually developed with a method from one of his competitors, Dr. Toussaint, and that he often strayed from the scientific method and inoculated patients with vaccines never tired on animals before. If the hero of medicine, Pasteur, stooped to plagiarism and lying when there was no money in play, imagine what we can expect from researchers now that there are fortunes at stake!

Those of us who have been published in "prestigious peer reviewed" journals know the feeling of pride and satisfaction of reading your name on top of the article. I love research. I have had the opportunity to publish nine articles in Austrian, German, Mexican and American medical journals, an accomplishment that catapulted me to a higher echelon in the scientific hierarchy. It is easy to get trapped in the web of "publicationism." I continue researching but without the pressures of publication. I find a lot more satisfaction now searching for new natural and non-aggressive ways to help my patients. Academic researchers first engage in research for the love of the art, but they end up being forced to publish. In the scientific world, we call it "publish or perish." Publications are the oxygen writers breathe. Since most research is conducted in isolated laboratories, the temptation to manipulate findings and data is irresistible. Doing so is often the quick way to gain attention and recognition. Industrial researchers are not into publications, they guard their secrets well. Their motivation, purely and simply, is money.

I was not surprised when the professional ethics of scientists were placed in serious doubt in January 1988 when *60 Minutes* aired a show entitled "The Facts Were Fiction." This report had its origin in a government investigation of scientific fraud directed by the state representative from Michigan, John Bingel, and the National Bureau of Standards. The investigation evaluated a host of scientific publications. The investigators concluded that more than 50% of the articles published were useless because there was no existing evidence that the researchers adequately evaluated what they claimed to be evaluating. Questionnaires were sent to 31 groups of researchers, requesting the worksheets containing their data. Some 21 responded with the claim that they had lost their documents or that they had been "accidentally" destroyed. The reporters asserted that between 10% and 30% of the research was totally fictitious. One of the experts interviewed declared, "I would think twice before believing what I read in medical journals. It is fraudulent information."

Prominent, respectable people from a variety of circles plagiarize and alter data and results with the desire to inflate their personal prestige. Johann Bernouilli (1700-1782), credited with the development of integral and exponential calculus and the law of conservation of energy, stole the equations from his son. Not only did he steal them, he altered the data to make his son look like the plagiarizer. Incredible! The geocentric theory of Ptolomeo reigned for 1500 years without its author ever having carried out one observation. Newton manipulated his calculations on the speed of sound and the equinoxes so that he could formulate his theory of gravity. He never lifted a finger, and not because gravity overpowered him.

The financial future of many products, especially pharmaceuticals, depend on the outcome of the researchers. This encourages scientific fraud. Incentives for scientists at important universities like Harvard, MIT, and Yale include prestigious publications, international recognition, travel, scholarships and patent rights which ensure them riches, power and the ultimate possible - a Nobel Prize. To attain all this, universities provide them with super laboratories and the most promising students, who act as slaves.

Today, scientists who put all their effort into serving humanity are few and far between. If the ultimate goal was to heal the sick, more scientists would behave like Dr. Jonas Salk who, counter to the advice of his coworkers, refused to patent his anti-polio vaccine so that the whole world could own it. Prizes, medallions and remuneration have proven to be irresistible. Yet, human lives lie in the balance. Dr. Robert Gallo of the National Cancer Institute, in his quest for the Nobel Prize, insisted that his group, not the Pasteur Institute, had discovered the AIDS virus. Courts found the allegations of Gallo fraudulent, and the French won the dispute nine years later. It is my opinion that such incentives should disappear in order to preserve the purity of motives in all sciences, especially medicine.

How can government agencies protect us from dangerous medications if they depend on research conducted by an industry that has sold out? How can they depend on fraudulent scientists who fall prey to the lure of fame and fortune? The description of this phenomenon is masterfully done by Dr. Herbert M. Shelton in his book *Hygienic Review* in which he states, "Science is the ever subservient handmaiden of commercialism; and we should not be surprised by the fact that the scientists can find and have found justification, even if only fictional, for all the practices that are fostered by the commercial world for profit."

The majority of the world's population uses medications that have probably been evaluated by dishonest scientists, and approved by government officials who dance to the music of money. The words of Linnaeus in his *Diaeta Naturalis* (Natural Diet, 18th century) ring true when he says, "to live dependent on medicine is to live hideously." Such words have never before taken on such depth of meaning as now, when the majority of human beings suffer from one disease or another, and when so many people depend on medication to keep them going each day. The most prescribed drugs are tranquilizers, sleeping pills, high blood pressure drugs, arthritic pain killers and antibiotics, all of which are consumed in industrial quantities. Billions of these pills are sold annually by drugstores.

The Consequences of the System

Although most of the information is not within the reach of the general public, those charged with keeping watch over public health, especially the FDA, have had big setbacks. The following cases will serve as a few examples of their blunders:

- The fallibility of the strict scientific method was put on display by the famous Thalidomide incident. Ingested by pregnant women to combat nausea, it produced severe deformities in their offspring. Around 1500 babies suffered the miserable consequences (*Lancet*).

- Another classic example is that of DES (diethylstilbestrol, a synthetic female hormone), which was used extensively from the 1940s to the 1970s, in spite of the fact that it had been shown by Dr. Lakasana from Paris in 1938 to cause cancer in rats. Thirty years later, the daughters of those who took DES showed an extraordinarily high incidence of vaginal, cervical and breast cancer, as well as liver damage, and their children suffered congenital deformities. These grave secondary effects persisted for two generations. In 1971, Dr. Arthur L. Herbst of Harvard University reported that not only was it not useful for the illness for which it was prescribed (antiabortives), but it was carcinogenic and teratogenic as well. But according to Robert F. Mendelsson, it was still prescribed as a "day after" contraceptive and to stop the flow of breast milk. It may surprise you to know that DES is still prescribed today.

- One of the antibiotics frequently prescribed by internists and surgeons is Flagyl. Although definitive and clinical evidence of its carcinogenic quality are irrefutable, there is no indication that authorities plan to withdraw it from the market.

- The Smith Kline Company put on sale a drug to treat hypertension called Selecrine after compliance with the FDA's rigorous norms. It was on sale from May 1979 to January 1980. This drug caused 36 deaths, and liver and kidney damage in a host of others. The laboratory denied that there was any relationship between these cases and the product, but the scientists who invented the drug were declared responsible for not reporting the evidence of risk of liver and kidney damage to the FDA, and the laboratory lost its case.

- In 1962, a drug for reducing cholesterol called Triparanol was withdrawn from the market when it was discovered that it caused a great many side effects, including cataracts.

- In 1993, a medicine called Felbatol which controlled epileptic seizures was put on the market, but it produced dangerous side effects.Twenty-one patients out of

100,000 developed a rare blood deadly disease called aplastic anemia. Four people have died.

• Reserpine, used to combat high blood pressure, continues to be used although it increases the incidence of breast cancer by 300%. It can also cause lethargy, nasal congestion, fatigue, cloudy vision, headaches, vertigo, sleep disorders and anxiety. It can cause gastrointestinal disorders like nausea, vomiting and diarrhea.

• I have already mentioned that among the drugs most prescribed are the ones used to combat high blood pressure. Hypertension develops in poorly nourished men and women under stress. Talk about market opportunity!. Merck produces one of the most popular, with annual sales of about one billion dollars. It may be that the anti-hypertension drugs contribute to bringing down your blood pressure but they do not reduce the mortality from heart attacks or embolism (blood clots). What does this mean? Patients who take these medications have the same mortality index as those who don't take them. Besides being an unnecessary cost, they produce headaches, nausea, and impotence.

• Not even the children are free of risk. Every day more cases of hyperactivity and ADD are being found among children. Dexedrin, Cylert, Ritalin, and Tofranil are prescribed for them. Parents don't know that these medications can damage the brain, sometimes permanently, or that they can solve their children's problems by making simple changes in their diet. Junk food is the main cause of behavioral problems in children. The negative effects of these medications are: high blood pressure, nervousness, and sleeplessness, as well as disturbed growth. Children show less disposition to respond to stimuli, they lose their sense of humor and become apathetic. They do not learn better at school, on the contrary, they act like zombies.

After a century of searching for "magic bullets," the dream of doing away with infections has not been realized. One hundred years after Koch discovered the microbe causing cholera, the World Health Organization declared that that devastating disease had been eradicated. But Cholera reappeared in the decade of the eighties and nineties. As for Tuberculosis, one third of the world still suffers from it and more people die from it than from any other disease. In 1992, the World Health Organization declared it a world health emergency of the first order. If at times we doctors have felt we had the power to defeat epidemics, today's perspective is distressing. Germs have become adept at developing resistance to antibiotics. In some cases, they have developed the ability to produce an enzyme that destroys antibiotics. The following chart will give an idea of the failure of medicine and the pharmaceutical industry to arrest infections.

The World's Deadliest Scourges

Infectious Disease	Cause	Annual Deaths
Acute Respiratory Infections (mostly pneumonia)	Bacterial or Viral	4,300,000
Diarrheal Diseases	Bacterial or Viral	3,200,000
tubercolosis	Bacterial	3,000,000
Hepatitis B	Viral	1,500,000
Malaria	Protozoan	1,000,000
Measles	Viral	880,000
Neonatal Tetanus	Bacterial	600,000
AIDS	Viral	550,000
Pertussis (Whoping Cough)	Bacterial	360,000

Source: *World Health Organization*

The pharmaceutical industry leaves nothing to chance. It relies on a team of experts to constantly visit doctors and enlighten them with incontrovertible scientific studies that prove the effectiveness of their products. As the newspaper USA Today noted, "In the United States, the pharmaceutical industry invests an average of ten billion dollars a year promoting its pharmaceuticals." How much will these investments yield in revenue? Let's take the case of Valium, the number one prescription drug in the United States, which is prescribed for an estimated sixty million people annually. Imagine the profit! These prescription narcotics (valium and others), kill more people than those distributed by drug dealers. In the United States, 30,000 people die annually from adverse reactions to narcotics, licit and illicit. In 1995, 7800 *people* (26%) were victims of the Mafia, the other 22,200 *patients* (74%), of the board-certified Mafi... excuse me, medical doctors!

The owners and directors of pharmaceutical corporations often fail to recognize or respect ethical and legal barriers when their interests are threatened. On January 6, 1994, Copley pharmaceutical, one of the largest producers of generic drugs, was faced with the embarrassment of recalling their anti-asthmatic drug, Albuterol, from drugstores. More than 10,000 patients had complained about severe reactions to this medication. The FDA received reports that more than 400 people, mainly children, had died as a result of taking contaminated Albuterol due to failure in the production process.

The company produced unflawed reports to the FDA, but some employees testified that the reports were manipulated and falsified. The FDA withdrew the medication from the market. To date, the company has not been punished. Since Copley Pharmaceutical's Albuterol was "withdrawn" from the market, 27,000 patients, unbeknown to the ruling, continued to buy it, and 37,000 new patients were started! How is this possible? Let me explain. When the FDA "withdraws" a product from the market, the laboratory must suspend production. However, drug stores are not legally obligated to stop selling it until their inventory and that of the wholesalers has been sold out. How considerate of the FDA!

Pressured by the public in 1972, the FDA began to evaluate over-the-counter drugs, especially those of doubtful effectiveness. The immense job of reviewing 2,486 therapeutic

preparations with 875 active ingredients has been very tedious, according to a reporter for U.S. News and World Report. More than twenty years later, only 70% had been evaluated. Many are a real threat to the public but few have been
"withdrawn." One of them, sulfate of quinine (used to control cramps), was withdrawn from the market by the FDA
because there was no sufficient evidence the drug produced
any therapeutic benefit, but there were an alarming number
of reports of severe adverse reactions, including sixteen
deaths. Yet, the product was in drug stores for more than
eighteen years before the FDA took action.

Lamentably, the FDA still has not reviewed 30% of the over-
the-counter drugs. It will take them many more years, but
these are not so toxic and that's why they don't need a prescription. Right? When will they reevaluate the real toxic
ones, those that require a prescription? In the rare cases
when the FDA has had to withdraw a product from the market because it was proven to be ineffective or dangerous, it
has only done so because the media has managed to get hold
of the information or the families of the many victims sue.

However, the pharmaceutical industry continues to look for
new horizons, either with new products or with brilliantly
innovative ideas. A supremely lucrative idea is to produce a
drug, banned in the USA, in their international franchises
where the health officials are not aware of the problem or

easily persuaded by bribes. Should companies be allowed to treat people of such countries as an inferior species? For example, Buscapine was prohibited in the United States because it was considered extremely noxious. Its side effects are hives, upper gastric pain, nausea, diarrhea, jaundice, and shock. However, in Mexico, dispensing it has never been prohibited since, in Mexico, "life is cheap." How many drugs do you suppose have been registered, which have hidden side effects that manifest themselves long after the drugs are ingested. The numbers are frightening.

Who Will Protect US?

It's too bad that the Society for the Prevention of Cruelty to Animals (SPCA) protects its animals more effectively than doctors protect people. In the United States, this movement, which is dedicated to the protection of animals, is seriously blocking the research of the pharmaceutical industry. Thanks to its tenacity, the movement has managed to save the Ginea Pigs. Bravo! Its influence has gone to ridiculous extremes. For example, in every film where animals are used, take note of a legend that appears at the end of the credits which states "In this film, the physical integrity of no animal has been exposed." I agree that mice must be protected, but because of such pressures research with animals has "gone south." Studies are still conducted using animals, but only in underdeveloped countries which are outside the jurisdiction of the

SPCA. Shortcuts save money, and with the record of the pharmaceutical industry, I don't doubt for a single moment that many studies usually made with animals are now being made with humans.

Incredibly, when the authorities of the FDA prohibit the sale of some products, like pesticides, for their toxicity, they only prohibit its distribution in the United States, but not their production. As an example, chemical companies ship to Mexico and other South American countries, pesticides like DDT and others that can't be used on American soil because of their carcinogenic quality. I agree that the responsibility of the public health services of this world are limited when their representatives have been deceived by the industry, but where is the justice that absolves them when the data concerning the dangers of a product is overwhelming, as they are on these pesticides and some pharmaceuticals? Well, Americans get their DDT back in the low cost produce they import from underdeveloped countries.

The FDA gives license to produce carcinogenic preservatives for junk foods, alcohol, and thousands of other items. Smoking cigarettes, for example, in the United States alone kills 419,000 people annually, mainly through cardiovascular disease and cancer. I imagine that the government's argument is that everyone is responsible for their own actions. Of course! Forget about the more than 30,000 that die from secondary smoking. But why then is heroine, which kills only 5,000 people a year in the United States, prohibited? In no way am I proposing that a drug like heroin be approved for general use, but this does demonstrate that the criteria of the health agencies is biased, illogical, and manipulated by the economic giants. Can we trust an authority that approves "convenience" products such as preservatives for fast foods, fake calorie-free fats, sweets laden with chemicals, pesticides, etc.?

Why aren't natural products promoted? There is a huge discrepancy in the attitude of health authorities when it comes to such laxity in the control of noxious chemical substances, as we have already highlighted, and their strict criteria for the authorization of nutritional supplements, whose beneficial effects have been demonstrated by scientific means. We, the doctors who work with alternative treatments, have witnessed the good results obtained with such therapies. Incredible, but Victor Hugo, a century ago, in his book *Things of the Infinite*, admonished us, "Science says the first word in everything and the last word in nothing." How do we explain this? From my personal point of view, the last word in everything is spoken by money.

First, I should limit the spectrum of responsibility. The developing countries (3rd world) unconditionally accept the resolutions of those who dictate (1st World) the guidelines to be followed. For example, in countries like mine, American chemical products and pharmaceuticals are automatically approved by our authorities because of the expansive and expensive investigations carried out by America's distinguished and ethical institutions. Oh, but don't try to import to the US pharmaceutical products approved by the health departments from our countries. Even though Mexico has the capability of doing such procedures, when the product gets to the FDA (this will happen as often as the Halley's comet comes to visit), every step has to be repeated!

The cost of registering a drug in the United States is astronomical. In order to comply with all the prerequisites imposed by the FDA, any one seeking to obtain approval or registration of a drug has to have incredible resources. It takes about 12 years to complete all the lab, animal and human trials by a host of teams. In the process the company or institution will spend an average of 250 million dollars for each drug. After all is done, you may be rejected! Making drugs is difficult. This absurd and complicated process was suggested by the pharmaceutical industry with the objective of protecting the end consumer. Really? The reality of the matter is that this expensive "show" is designed to protect this "major-league" industry. In 1990, the general accounting office of the United States reported that the top pharmaceutical companies showed earnings up to three times larger, on the average, than the other most profitable companies in America. The money comes mostly from insurance companies, but it hits hard on the economy of the sick.

The FDA process of approval "muscles" the small competi-
tor out of the game. Many aspiring laboratories of biotech-
nology like Immunogen, Bioprocess Technologies,
Halometrics, and some two hundred others failed because of
these strict and expensive norms.

Anyone who has a drop of intelligence would not spend 48
thousand dollars a day for twelve years to prove the therapeutical value of broccoli or garlic, so that the FDA gives you
permission to make claims and write prescriptions for it and
then not protect your investment with a patent because natural products are of public domain. Any small time lab would
be able to take advantage of your 250 million dollar project.
Up to now, no one has had such love for humanity. Now, if it
was to save the street dogs of the third world maybe the SPCA
would front the money. I believe that we should protect all
species in our world. I admire the activists that fight for animal rights, but maybe we should all fight first for the prevention of cruelty to humans.

The Benefits of Technology for Health

The technological revolution of the twentieth century, as
unbelievable as it may seem, has had an insignificant impact on the health of the general public. In reality, it has had
a negative effect. The "takeoff" of medical science began
with the control of disease through the use of antibiotics. But, though this and other accomplishments

have been important, as mentioned before, diseases have only been partially controlled. In spite of everything, including our sophisticated machines, germs have their own agenda for making fools of us. The war on common disease continues to be a thorn in the side of scientists. Cancer therapies are a failure, no cure has been found for arthritis, diabetes, multiple sclerosis, and many other diseases. Often, the treatments for these afflictions only address the symptoms. Furthermore, the treatments have side effects that are sometimes worse than the diseases. For example, the non-steroid anti-inflammatory substances, while offering temporary relief for the symptoms of arthritis, cause severe gastritis, peptic ulcers, and bone decalcification. These side effects cause the hospitalization of 170,000 annually, and between ten thousand and twenty thousand deaths.

Help from the North

For centuries, we have put our faith in doctors and medical science. Should we really put ourselves blindly into their hands? The confidence we have given to medical science has its roots in the conviction that research is carried out in university and governmental institutions unlinked to economic and political interests. We believe that their discoveries and advances are motivated by a concern for social well-being and nothing else. Many are convinced that scientific research remains pure and unadulterated.

The best example is the group research conducted in the famed National Institutes of Health in the United States (NIH). They are a division of the Department of Health and Human Resources. Their proposed function is to better public health and provide research into the causes and prevention of disease. At present, the NIH relies on eleven establishments. Among them are the National Institute for Allergies and Infectious Diseases; the National Institute for Heart, Lungs, and Blood; Institutes for Ophthalmology, Neurology, Odontology, and several others. Yet, the most prominent is the National Cancer Institute (NCI), which, different from the other eleven, answers directly to the Secretary of Health and not to the Director of the NIH. These very famous "campuses," thus named for their similarity to traditional universities, are nested among the lush meadows of Maryland, near Washington, D.C. They are surrounded by lawns as carefully groomed as those of a golf course. The annual budget of the NIH is 6.5 billion dollars. Since the eighties, 1.5 billion dollars of that budget belongs to the NCI. The rest is divided between the other eleven institutes. This budget is the largest of any research institute in the entire world.

Fearsome Enemy

There is no doubt that the struggle against cancer is the greatest challenge that medical science has ever faced. There is no other disease to which more money is devoted, or to which scientists dedicate more hours of study. Since the twenties, vast resources have been invested in the search for a cure, and since that time we have been hearing reports of valuable discoveries. In 1955, the NCI established the Chemotherapy National Service Center (CNSC) appropriating 25 million dollars to "promote" this anti-cancer treatment since "it was demonstrated" that chemotherapy "proved to be an effective treatment for cancer patients, not only in the United States, but around the world." Why, if it is so effective, is so much money needed to promote it? Two years later, Lawrence Rockerfeller encouraged us with a report stating the progress in oncological research, declaring in *Reader's Digest* (1957), "There is for the first time the smell of victory in the air." An article filling an entire page in the New York Times (1969) stated that "a cancer cure is at hand," predicting the arrival of a definitive treatment by 1976.

In December of 1971, president Richard M. Nixon, in response to the call of Elmer Bobst of the American Cancer Society (ACS), signed the National Cancer Act. So, the government of the United States, along with the ACS, officially declared "war on cancer." Dr. Vincent T. De Vita, director of the NCI, promised a victory and the reduction of the death rate for cancer in half in a decade, if sufficient funds weregiven. Five years later, in the annual assembly where the directors of the president's national cancer panel give their progress report to the president of the United States, no positive results could be given. No progress had been made. In 1980, the NCI felt obliged to report that very little ground had been gained, and its members were fearful of losing face.

Curiously, in 1983 the NCI reported to the media that significant progress had been made in the war against cancer. "In the past 20 years, critical care medicine has emerged as a specialty in its own right, paralleling improving trends in cancer treatment. Cancer surgery has become less radical, radiotherapy more precise and less toxic because the normal treatment volume has become smaller, and chemotherapy less empirical, more effective and less toxic. More cancer patients are alive and well as a result." said Dr. De Vita.

The comments of Dr. De Vita never cease to dumbfound me. Though it is true that the advances in trauma medicine have been miraculous, impressively diminishing death rates in accident victims and those with surgical emergencies, the death rate of patients with cancer has never stopped rising. I agree that surgery and radiation have been moderated, not because medical doctors are convinced that they are more effective, but because they have been disillusioned by the pessimistic results and toxicity of radical treatment. Even more curious is the comment that chemotherapy has become less empirical. By his statement, Dr. De Vita publicly accepted the fact that chemotherapy was lacking scientific foundation. His statement would not be so surprising were it not for the fact that the most severe criticism directed against the "empirism" of alternative therapies. The final statement is a flagrant lie. The results have not been good. In 1972 about 330, 000 patients died of cancer in the USA, according to De Vita's promise, by 1982 the number should have dropped to 165, 000. In spite of an overabundance of funds, the rate surpassed the 400, 000 mark.

In May of 1986, Dr. John C. Bailar III of Harvard Univesity and Elaine Smith of the University of Iowa published in the New England Journal of Medicine an "atomic bomb" against orthodox oncology. They concluded that the advances left much to be desired in view of the fact that the most common forms of cancer remained uncontrollable. They insisted that the scientific world reconsider the present guiding principles of cancer research, along with their application. In comparison to cardiovascular diseases, where a downward trend in the death rate is evident, the death rate of cancer patients continues to rise. Dr. Bailar III and his team concluded that they "were losing the war against cancer," and that "substantial progress in the understanding of the nature and attributes of cancer" had not led to "a reduction of the incidents of mortality." Therefore, they asserted that "the most promising areas of cancer research are those of prevention rather than treatment."

In spite of the prestige of these authors, their respective universities, and the strength of their argument, their wise recommendations went in one ear and out the other as far as the scientific community was concerned. Twenty billion dollars and 25 years after Nixon's initiative, the outlook for the effective treatment of cancer is discouraging. 1996 saw the highest figures in cancer history, both in incidence and death. Tom Beardsley from Scientific American, zooms into the problem: "The obviously illusory comments of the NCI have only increased the impatience of the critics." In 1984, under Dr. De Vita, the NCI theatrically announced the "reachable" goal of reducing the death rate by 50 percent in 20 years (1980-2000). In other words, they asserted that by the beginning of the 21st century only 245,000 people would die from cancer annually. Compare this prediction with reality. In 1985, (graph needs to be corrected)over 485,000 people died from cancer.

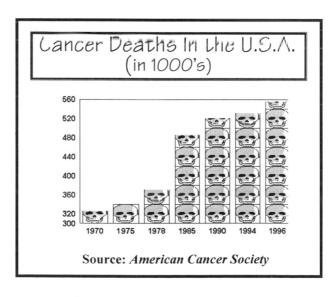

Cancer Deaths In the U.S.A.
(in 1000's)

Source: *American Cancer Society*

In 1996, the ACS predicted 555,000 deaths, but some statisticians concluded the actual number was close to 700,000 people that died from malignancies. Could it be that their poor nutritional habits have affected their mathematical skills?

A depressing picture of "approved" treatments against cancer (surgery, radiation, and chemotherapy) is revealed in an evaluation made by the ACS. In their annual publication of *Cancer Facts and Figures* for 1996, they show virtually no improvement among the most frequently appearing tumors in the last 60 years, with the exception of cancer of the stomach and cervix.

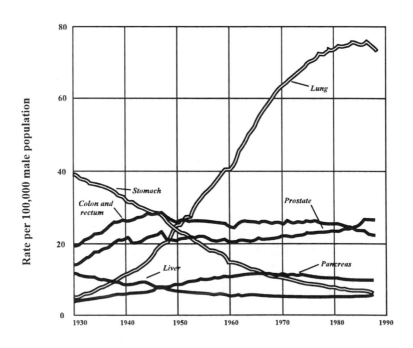

The improvements in the death rates of people suffering from these two malignancies is an enigma; the failure of treatments isn't. In the case of stomach cancer it is conjectured that the improvements are due to better hygiene, healthier foods, and the advent of endoscopy, which detects gastric diseases in the early stages. However, treatments for this type of cancer are a complete failure and have not contributed to the improvement in the mortality rate.

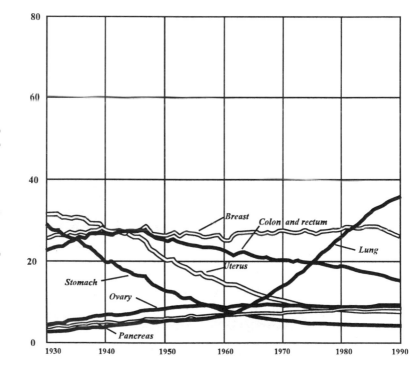

Neither is the treatment approved for cervical-uterine cancer responsible for the improvement in the death rate. In fact, the downward slope in the graph indicates that improvement began a long time before modern scientific advances, like radiation therapy, were introduced. The improvement is due to a simple invention in 1928 by Dr. Papanicolau, who created the test which detects cervical cancer - the "PAP SMEAR." As hard as it may be to believe, the FDA wouldn't approve this test until 1940. Imagine how many women died needlessly because of this terminal delay. Yet, no one claimed responsibility for this negligence.

In all the other malignancies graphed, statistical records indicate that the "enormous scientific advances" have not helped patients survive. On the contrary, where the malignancies are treated with aggressive remedies, the death rates are incredibly high. Even if the patients survive, the quality of life they endure afterwards is impaired, often permanently. The death rate of people suffering from pulmonary cancer has literally exploded. This is due to the fact that many women began smoking cigarettes in the 1960's as a result of the women's liberation movement. Why woman decided to lower their standards and act like men is a mystery to me. Now, lung cancer is the number one killer in women, the same as in men! I'm sure this was not the equality they were searching for.

Women, for reasons unknown, seem more vulnerable to cigarette smoke and consequently more susceptible to lung cancer than men.

All Smoke But No Fire

The evolution and development of products in various branches of industry have been impressive. No one today would buy a 10 year old computer, in America not even a 6 month old! The new computers offer so many advantages that the obsolete one would soon seem like a hindrance rather than a help. In most of the branches of medicine significant changes have also taken place. For example there are plastic catheters so sophisticated that they can remain inside the body for years. Those that could only be left in place for a few weeks have been abandoned, even if the patient only needs on for a week. The evolution of antibiotics has made past versions obsolete. However, in the treatment of cancer there has been no substantial change. Even though technological developments have been applied to these treatments, technology has only served as a cosmetic improvement. In the meantime, we continue to fight cancer with the same weapons (surgery, radiation, and chemotherapy), although more sophisticated. The medical community continues to re-deal the same cards over and over again.

In 1994, the cover of the April 25 edition of Time magazine proclaimed, "New discoveries promise improved therapies and hope in the war against cancer." This kind of statement not only rings false but, in view of the evidence, it is downright offensive. The article refers to "discoveries" related to genetic mutations associated with the formation of specific tumors. Unfortunately, the therapeutic application of these discoveries remains in the far distant future. On this level of investigation, scientists are delving into the heart of creation. The risks are enormous and the consequences might be worse than the disease. Besides, the discoveries are hardly "new." Scientists have been working in these areas since the 1960's and their accomplishments have been minimal. After watching the scientific community spend exorbitant amounts on an unsuccessful 30 year research project to find a cure, I have come to conclude. (as any kindergartner could), that prevention is the best medicine. Yet, the budget for prevention research ridiculously small!

The Science of Sabotage

In other branches of modern science and industry, obsolescence is an every day occurrence and new processes replace the old even if they are working; things have to improve! Regarding the cancer issue, the governmental authorities, scientific community, and pharmaceutical monopolies have placed serious obstacles in the path of new ideas. Alternative therapies, many of which have been proven effective, have been ridiculed, pushed aside, and prohibited. These therapies do not deteriorate the patients quality of life. It is well known that patients suffering from many malignancies live longer and better if the orthodox treatments (surgery, radiation, and chemotherapy) are not applied.

In 1969, Dr. Hardin James of the University of California at Berkeley reported at an ACS conference, that patients not subjected to the aggressive conventional therapies had a longer life expectancy, occasionally up to four times as long. In 1986, Dr. Bailar III and Elaine Smith reported that patients with lung cancer who were not treated have a longer life expectancy and enjoy a better quality of life than those who receive treatment. In 1988, Dr. Abel reported that, in an experiment with patients suffering from pancreatic cancer, those who received the placebo treatment instead of the real treatment lived longer and better. It seems like common sense, in the face of these testimonies, to conclude that more doctors should prescribe placebos. Unfortunately, to do so outside the confines of an experimental setting could land a physician in jail. Not uncommon in the medical world. Bailar III and Smith, upon evaluating the results of cancer therapies between 1950 and 1980, rated them to be a "qualified failure." When asked why he used the word "qualified," he replied, "Because the studies of treatments were done only by qualified scientists." Eight years later, a reevaluation published in the Scientific American (1994) reported that the mortality rate for people with cancer continued to climb. These men and women are not joking when they assert that treatment methods and the direction of the research must change. A serious research group needs to study and publish, in a peer reviewed journal, the profound meaning of "barking up the wrong tree."

The "Scientific" Basis of Cancer Treatment

Surgery

The general criterion for the surgical treatment of cancer were established around the turn of the century, starting with breast cancer. At the end of the 19th century, the important thing in surgery, the barbers domain, was the speed with which it was performed, since the surgeon operated without anesthesia or antibiotics. In the last quarter of the 19th century, the following changes took place in regard to surgical procedure:

- It was discovered that ether could be used as an anesthesia.
- Joseph Lister discovered that infection could be reduced by eliminating bacteria.
- Surgeons began washing their hands to reduce post-operative infection.
- Surgeons began washing their instruments more frequently to reduce infection.
- Antiseptics were introduced.
- In Germany, techniques and instruments were developed to control blood loss.

These factors set the stage for surgery as it is practiced today. During this period, William Halsted, considered to be the father of surgery in the United States, made his debut. Halsted entered Columbia University's medical program in 1874 at the age of 22. He subsequently continued his studies for two years in the great hospitals of Germany and Austria. In Halsted's professional development Rudolph Virchow, a German pathologist, archeologist, and anthropologist, played a major role. Virchow was also known as the pope of German medicine.

In Halsted's day, breast cancer was treated either by extricating the tumor itself or by removing the entire breast. Halsted visualized the disease as growing by spreading its "tentacles" far and wide. In Germany, students of Virchow had been told that carcinogenic cells were not spread through the blood stream. Cancer of the liver and lungs, they believed, arrived directly through these "tentacles" to the organs. The theory of "centrifugal dissemination" became the foundation of oncological surgery. Therefore, the maximum possible amounts of tissue, in which such "tentacles" might be hidden, had to be removed.

Based on such a theory, Halsted expanded the techniques he had learned in Germany and began to practice radical mastectomy, an operation that involved the removal of the whole breast and much of the surrounding tissue. For this reason it was necessary to do the following:

- Remove all of the infected breast.
- Remove the adjacent muscles of the chest.
- Remove all the lymph nodes in the armpit.

Halsted's radical mastectomy procedure was widely accepted in the United States and Europe. Halsted once stated that only three of every fifty patients had recurrences, a statement that was clearly not based on factual evidence. The great ability and discipline of Halsted succeeded in turning his approach into a teaching model for surgery in the United States. The philosophy and technique of radical surgery for breast cancer was soon applied to other kinds of malignancies. For example, surgeons of the head and neck had developed the "commando" operation, in which the jaw bone, the muscles of the neck, and the blood vessels with their lymphatic ganglia were removed. Obviously, such a procedure left the patient mutilated. The name "commando" is attributed to a technique used by soldiers in World War II to decapitate an enemy soldier.

In 1910, James Ewing of New York Memorial Hospital published evidence that cancerous cells are spread to distant organs from the original tumor via the blood stream (metastasis). So it was that the theory of centrifugal dissemination of Virchow and Halsted fell. Metastasis and reoccurrence constituted a surgeon's nightmare, and still do. Although it was proven that radical surgery didn't do away with the tentacles of tumor activity, surgeons blamed themselves for not removing enough tissue. Many surgeons respond in the same way today. As a consequence, they constantly developed even more radical surgical techniques. To date, they continue to perform these drastic surgeries without any "scientific" foundation. In 1943, Frank Adair reported that 63 patients in Sloan Kettering Memorial Hospital who chose conservative surgery lived just as long as those who chose radical surgery. Yet, in spite of this evidence, Adair's results were suffocated by the establishment, out of fear of rejection and to please his superiors he said "it would be disastrous if we took a step backward."

During the 1950's, a group of surgeons began to question Halsted's ideas. George Crile of the Cleveland Clinic, a practitioner of radical surgery, found out about results obtained by a British surgeon by the name of Geoffrey Keynes in the practice of conservative surgery. Crile persuaded his colleagues to allow him to follow the conservative focus. Crile became the first physician in the United States to undergo a prospective clinical trial with conservative surgery for breast cancer. The majority of his patients received partial mastectomies. That is to say, he removed all of the tumor and an ample margin of healthy tissue. Crile's results were comparable to those obtained by radical surgery. Contrary to Adair, he chose to expose the establishment, and was censored as an extremist, just an inch away from being labeled a quack.

The breach between the defenders of radical surgeries and those of the conservative type began to widen. The very mention of conservative methodology fed more fuel to the fire of the self-styled "experts." Surgery became even more aggressive, Halsted's mastectomy was amended and expanded; besides removing the entire breast, chest muscles, and lymph nodes of the axillae, the "amended mastectomy" removed all the lymphatic ganglia under the sternum. This left the thorax of the patient looking like a washboard, because the ribs were now only covered by the skin.

The big shot surgeons of Columbia and the Mayo Clinic constantly pressed for more extensive surgeries, inventing the "super-radical mastectomy." In this procedure, the clavicle was fractured and the first rib removed in order to allow doctors to more easily cut out more tissue. Fortunately, this procedure was soon abandoned due to its disastrous results, much of which were attributable to the psychological impact of the mutilation.

Since patients continued to die, in spite of this "tumoral unloading," unfortunately for the patient the treatment of breast cancer acquired a multidisciplinary twist. This took the form of a committee consisting of a surgeon, radiation specialist, and an oncologist who planned the treatment strategy to be used in "attacking" the cancer. The multidisciplinary focus continues to this day. For example, chemotherapy may be given before surgery to reduce the size of the tumor, or it may be given after surgery as a "preventative" treatment. There are numerous strategic variations; the patients travel from doctor to doctor exhausting treatment options, but these interventions that *may* reduce local recurrence, also reduce the quality of the patient's life. None of them increase the patient's chances for survival. After diagnosis, patients are threatened and pained enough by the cancer, then they are made to suffer radical surgery, later they are tortured with radiation and chemothcrapy.

During the 1960s, there was a resurgence of enthusiasm for conservative breast surgery. Physicians leaned toward less aggressive surgery and literal preservation of the breast, which meant that only the tumor was removed. This procedure was referred to as a local extrication, tumorectomy, lumpectomy, or nodulectomy. When it was necessary to take away a part of the breast, it was called a partial mastectomy Baclesse studied the experiences of 100 patients treated with lumpectomy and radiation between 1937 and 1953 and concluded that the results of conservative surgery were as good as those obtained by radical surgery.

In 1964, the first major scientific study of conservative surgery for breast cancer was initiated. The study compared the removal of the tumor (local extrication) coupled with low doses of radiation therapy against radical mastectomy.

It concluded that the life expectancy of patients treated with conservative surgery was the same as those who underwent radical mastectomies. This study, which was carried out in Guy's Hospital in London, was severely criticized and the conservative movement suffered a costly setback.

It was at this point that George Crile of the Cleveland Clinic decided to take part in the debate. In 1965, Crile published a record of his experiences and continued to insist that conservative treatment was safe and effective. At Harvard University, Oliver Cope, who practiced conservative surgery, wrote about his experiences to the New England Surgical Study (1967), but was denied publication in their magazine. This was evidence of the fear that a conservative treatment might alter the status quo. In spite of the opposition from the proponents of radical surgery, the conservative forces began to gain influence and generated support from others who opposed radical surgery. In 1963, some physicians sought a balance between the two positions and suggested the removal of the breast and the armpit lymph nodes without removing the pectoral muscles. Although this made the procedure more difficult, the results were more aesthetically pleasing. This method has been referred to as a "modified" radical mastectomy. It has been well accepted internationally, but it still involves the often unnecessary mutilation of the body.

Halstead's Hypotheses	The Findings of the NSABP
1.Tumor cells are only spread by direct extension and they spread in an orderly manner.	1.Cancer cells do not follow an orderly pattern, but break away from the tumor and travel through the lymph nodes.
2.The network of lymph nodes act as barriers to the passage of tumor cells, and are not involved in the spread of the disease.	2.Lymphatic lymph nodes do not impede the passage of tumor cells, but often aid the spread of the cancer. Their invasion is an indication of a weak immune system.
3.Tumors grow and spread on their own and the patient's condition does not influence this process in any way.	3.The condition of the patient directly influences every aspect of the tumor's progress.
4.The bloodstream does not play an important role in the spread of cancer cells.	4.The blood stream acts as a "highway" for cancer cells to spread throughout the body.
5.Tumors will remain isolated and encapsulated inside the body for a long time.	5.Cancer cells begin to circulate at a very early stage. Cancer is a systemic disease.
6.The kind of surgical treatment is very important to the survival of the patient.	6.Local treatment has little effect on a patient's chances for survival.

In 1957, Bernard Fisher of the University of Pittsburgh organized a multi-institutional group called National Surgical Adjuvant Breast Project (NSABP). This group was dedicated to the study of the several aspects of mammary cancer. Fisher formed this group because he was not convinced of the validity of Halsted's hypothesis.

This group soon began to refute Halsted's hypothesis, through a series of studies. The NSABP successfully refuted many of the ideas of Halsted's hypothesis. No institution and no individual has contributed more to the understanding of cancer than Dr. Fisher and the NSABP.

According to Halsted, the removal of the lymph nodes is absolutely necessary. Yet, the validity of his prescription has been the focus of heated discussion at international oncological conferences. An important study was done by the NSABP which concentrated on the treatment of the lymph nodes. Surgeons treated more than a thousand women with mammary cancer. None of these women had palpable lymphatic glands in the armpit. The patients were divided into three groups: patients treated by radical mastectomy, patients treated by simple mastectomy with radiation therapy on the lymph nodes, and patients treated by simple mastectomy without radiation to the ganglia. Approximately 18 % of the patients treated experienced cancerous spread to the lymph nodes. The surprising thing was that the survival rate was the same for all three groups. Therefore, it became apparent that there was no advantage gained when the lymph nodes were removed by surgery or treated with radiation. The myth, which was forwarded by proponents of radical surgery, was completely discredited. The NSABP concluded that surgeons can leave the lymph nodes alone, even when they harbor cancerous cells, without jeopardizing the patient's chances for survival.

By the 1970s, breast cancer treatment was the main topic of discussion in oncological circles. In 1972, the prestigious magazine British Medical Journal affirmed that there was "more controversy about the management of breast cancer than of any other aspect of tumoral therapy." Supporters of conservative therapies concluded that recurrence was not eminent. Vera Peter of Toronto considered that, "although the rate of recurrence is significantly higher in patients treated with conservative surgery, their life expectancy is the same." It is true that 20 % of the patients treated with conservative surgery experience recurrences, but it is also true that they can be treated with another conservative operation. Although 20 % seems like a high percentage, remember that 80 % are spared a devastating operation that would severely reduce the quality of their lives. Spitalier of Marseilles, France, concluded in *Radiation Oncology* that recurrences are operable and do not appear to be associated with the lowering of life expectancy.

In 1970, John Stehlin of St. Joseph's Hospital in Houston began to treat patients with partial mastectomies and radiation therapy. In 1979, he published a record of his experiences with 79 women in *Surgery: Gynecology and Obstetrics*. His record demonstrated that conservative breast surgery is as effective as its radical counterpart.

As was to be expected, he was severely criticized by his colleagues. They set aside his conclusions and continued with the established surgical methods. In 1996, the ACS expected more than 180,000 women to develop breast cancer. The majority of those women were treated with mastectomy, but more than 20 medical centers around the United States initiated protocols calling for treatment by conservative surgery and radiation.

Since you can't blot out the sun with one finger, most prominent medical journals began to publish articles in which the central message asserted that patients treated with conservative surgery and radiation live as long as those treated with radical mastectomy. In 1985, the NSABP published the first results of a comparative study of conservative surgical treatments (simple mastectomy, lumpectomy with post-operative radiation therapy). The study concluded that patients treated with lumpectomy, the most conservative treatment of the three, lived as long as those who received one of the other two treatments. No other cancer has been as thoroughly studied as breast cancer. Yet, when the patient with breast cancer is given the option for conservative surgery, like lumpectomy, they express a preference for the radical approach. Unbelievable! Why? What happens is that surgeons will often present the conservative option as "risky," claiming that there is still insufficient data to support it as the best approach. As we come toward the close of the century, incredibly, radical surgery is still the favored approach for the treatment of breast cancer. Nevertheless, this approach is in the process of being modified and the conservative approach is gaining acceptance.

The innocuous behavior of recurring tumors is a mystery. Some surgeons think that leaving a few cancerous cells to roam about after surgery is a deadly mistake. Others believe that these cells simply turn into tumors that can be removed without threatening the life of the patient. Still, many leaders in the field of oncological surgery, either out of fear or arrogance, continue to demand that more studies be conducted before modifying the traditional treatments. How many patients will become the innocent victims of this irrational posturing? The same tendencies have also been observed in other types of tumors. For example, sarcomas are tumors that generally form from muscle or fat in the extremities. Treatment of them always consists of an extensive amputation followed by radiation therapy, with the object of reducing the incidence of recurrence. After reviewing the experiences of numerous hospitals, one concludes that "a reduction of local recurrence does not mean a betterment of average life expectancy in the long run." In other words, the frightening mutilations are entirely unnecessary. The same conclusions can be applied to melanoma a very aggressive skin cancer, which is generally treated with excessively radical surgery.

In 1992, George Crile, the pioneer of conservative surgery

in the United States, died of lung cancer. He had dedicated his life to protecting women from disfiguring surgery. Two decades before his death, his theories had been amply confirmed. Nevertheless, he never received recognition from the establishment. In his autobiography, *The Way It Was — Sex, Surgery, Treasure, and Travel — 1907-1987*, a note of sadness is heard. He said, "in retrospect it has been proved that most of what I said was correct. In spite of that, to my knowledge, not one of my critics has retracted a single one of their accusations. Neither was I elected to a post in the American Cancer Society, the American Medical Association, or any other reputable medical organization." How is it possible that 60 years after the discovery that tumors spread by means of the blood stream, we won't change our surgical criteria? What justification could we possibly have to continue mutilating people when scientific, clinical studies prove that such a course of action is absolutely unnecessary? The cruelty of surgery reached its peak in the 1970's, when it occurred to Dr. Theodore Miller of the Sloan Kettering Cancer Center that the preferable method of fighting pelvic cancer was a hemiocorporectomy. This was a surgery that bordered on the macabre. Everything below the rib cage was removed, making it necessary to perform a colostomy and nephrostomies so that the patient could defecate and urinate through the skin. Imagine the monsters such a surgery created! It is said that the operations were successful, but the patients died, though not from surgical complications because technological advances made such an outrage possible.

They died from emotional trauma because they weren't able to accept themselves in their sub-human condition. Fortunately, no surgeon has ever seen fit to remove the top half of a human being, though it would seem that we are not exempt from such a possibility. The results were as horrible as the surgery themselves, and these "butcher" jobs were abandoned. Thank God!

This terrible procedure was the straw that broke the camel's back and predisposed us to practice more conservative procedures. Curiously, but tragically, it was surgical excess (the hemiocorporectomy) that set us on the road to moderation. Finally, the shame failure brings, deteriorated the image of the oncological authorities, no longer could they block (so harshly) the advent of more conservative surgeries. There is very little difference between the oncology of the last century and the present one, because its main instrument continues to be the scalpel. Today, when tumors are found in the early stages, surgery is the only weapon considered effective. If the patient is not mutilated, surgery is also considered the least aggressive treatment.

Since 1965, my father, based on the studies of Crile and others, denounced these agressive procedures. Like others before him, he was strongly criticized, condemned as a "quack" and an ignoramous in oncology. Today, many surgeons continue to perform radical surgeries on mammary cancer, in spite of the fact that even the great men of oncological surgery have discovered for themselves that women respond very well to the less destructive procedures. Let's harbor no hope that they will give the credit of these discoveries to the "quacks" that pioneered such research. At first, the promoters of a new and revolutionary idea are villainized, then they are ridiculed and ostracized. When change is finally embraced as valuable, the people who acted as the sharpest opponents against it often take credit for the idea.

Sophisticated modern medicine has tried to convert the art of medicine into an exact science through technology and mechanization. Not to practice medicine as an art is a mortal offense to the Hippocratic Oath in the eyes of Dr. Ernesto Contreras Sr., founder of The Oasis of Hope Hospital. "Fantasy abandoned by reason produces monsters, but when united to it, is the mother of all art," once said Francisco Goya, a famous Spanish artist. I truly hope that we stop this monstrous medical practice.

Radiation: An Act of Desperation

Radiation therapy, in which we placed so much faith a few decades ago, has proven to be another medical blunder. Motivated by the desperation of failure, the radiation therapists dreamed up new ways of applying increasingly aggressive doses to their patients. They literally "burned" them, leaving many permanently disabled, without sparing them the temporary side effects of severe nausea, malaise, loss of appetite, and the loss of other functions. They went to the extreme of dosing the entire body with frightening results. The reaction to these most extreme measures was much the same as the reaction to the extreme surgical treatments like the hemiocorporectomy. The medical community cringed in horror, and reverted to more conservative treatments.

My brother, Dr. Ernesto Contreras Jr., an oncologist and radio-therapist said, after 25 years of medical practice, "It is really frustrating to see how little we have been able to achieve in oncology. The effectiveness of the treatment against cancer is doubtful. I have treated thousands of patients, most of them in the advanced stages of cancer, and I can't say that more than 15% of them had positive response to an orthodox treatment. Only another 25% received the benefit of a temporary remission, or a real alleviation of the devastation caused by the disease. Most of the remaining 60% felt only a slight reduction in pain. I can say that only in a few patients, quality of life was significantly prolonged by the aggressive treatments now available. On the other hand, I have to accept, in many cases, that the remedy was worse than the disease."

"I am convinced that the real and practical value of chemotherapy and radiation therapy is very limited to specific cases. As long as we are unable to find better treatments for the vast majority of patients with cancer, it is an obligation, not just an occupation, that oncologists and physicians dedicate their efforts toward the investigation of new and alternative treatments. Only then can we hope to find more effective, less aggressive and less toxic treatments. Only then can we hope to prolong the lives of cancer patients and maintain the quality of their lives as well."

"I don't believe that the great research centers of the world have the right to conduct cancer research alone. The history of medicine is filled with anecdotes of the humble researcher, without the assistance of outside resources, who seized the opportunity to make highly significant contributions to medicine. Personally, I have decided to leave almost all administration of chemotherapy to other oncologists and to turn my radiation therapy department over to other radiation therapists. I am also determined to consider no remedy to be ridiculous until it is shown to be such, after receiving ample opportunity to demonstrate its benefits."

Chemotherapy: A Fate Worse Than Death

Since nothing else has worked in the fight against cancer, it is no surprise that frustration drives chemotherapists to give increasingly more aggressive treatments, both in regard to dosage and variety of substances used. All oncologists know that chemotherapy is the most toxic and least effective treatment. However, something must be done for the patient, and often desperation makes chemotherapy seem like the only option. So the therapists continue to rely on this destructive treatment, which borders on the sadistic. In most cases, the patients will feel like they are dying. They experience nausea and vomiting so severe that they must be hospitalized to help them endure the side effects. The hair of most chemotherapy patients falls out. They lose their appetite and even their will to live. Many of my patients would rather die than continue with such therapy. They actually prefer to take their chances with cancer, than to suffer the experience of chemotherapy, because the therapy is viewed as a fate worse than death.

The summary of the results of chemotherapy was published by Dr. Ulrich Abel in his book *Chemotherapy for Advanced Epithelial Cancer*, in which he throws down one of the most solid pillars of orthodox oncology. The term "epithelial cancer" encompasses cancer of the lungs, breast, prostate, colon and other organs. Epithelial cancers are responsible for 80% of the deaths attributable to cancer in the industrialized world. During his 10 years as a statistician, Abel discovered that the method used for treating the most commonly occurring epithelial cancers has rarely been successful.

Such a judgment as this has a significant impact when we remember that Dr. Abel belongs to the establishment that prescribes such treatments. Each time more toxic chemotherapies are used to "prevent" cancer.

Abel affirms that there is no evidence that the vast majority of cancer treatments with cytotoxic drugs (chemotherapy) exert any kind of positive influence as far as life expectancy or quality of life are concerned. The "almost dogmatic belief in the efficacy of chemotherapy is generally based on false conclusion drawn from inaccurate data." Abel assures us that after interviews with many doctors "the criteria of oncologists" is "a surprising contradiction in communication directed to the public," since many oncologists acclaim the benefits of chemotherapy in their publications but would not take it if they had cancer themselves.

Dr. Heine H. Hansen, in a survey involving 118 doctors - many of them cancer specialists- was shocked to find that oncologists recommend to most patients experimental chemotherapy which experts in the field would not accept for themselves. The vast majority of doctors consider that most of the treatment options with more than two to six drugs were unacceptable treatment options if they themselves were to take part in the clinical trials (The Journal of Clinical Oncology, Nov. 1987).

The establishment insists that one of the beneficial effects of chemotherapy is that it prolongs life expectancy by five years. According to Dr. Abel, this claim is clearly false. There is only evidence that chemotherapy extends life in the case of small cell carcinoma of the lung. This improvement consists of a life extension of only three months. Three months of torture!

These are some of the findings Dr. Abel published regarding some cancers commonly treated with chemotherapy:

- Colon and Rectal Cancer: There is no evidence at all that chemotherapy prolongs the life of patients suffering these malignancies.
- Stomach cancer: No evidence of effectiveness.
- Pancreatic Cancer: The largest study was "completely negative." The patients who experienced prolonged life were those who did not receive chemotherapy.
- Bladder Cancer: Chemotherapy is often applied but is not effective. No prospective study has been made.
- Breast Cancer: There is no evidence that chemotherapy raises the chances for a patients survival. Its use is "ethically questionable."
- Ovarian Cancer: There is no direct evidence, but it might be worthwhile to research the use of platinum.
- Uterine and Cervical Cancer: There was no improve ment in the survival rate of those treated with chemotherapy.
- Cancer of the head and neck: There was no benefit to receiving chemotherapy in terms of survival. There was the occasional benefit of reduction of tumor size.

In the face of these facts, it is fitting to ask the source of the data that supports that chemotherapy is beneficial.

Cheating happened! It is true that sometimes these medications do, in effect, reduce tumor size, but this has no significant impact in regard to life extension, and almost always a monstrous disaster for the quality of life. As a matter of fact, the cancer sometimes comes back more aggressive than ever. Even though 99% of a tumor is eliminated, the resistant 1% is often made up of the most aggressive cells.

In spite of the illuminating report on chemotherapy by Dr. Abel, there does not seem to be any tendency within the medical world to use more conservative methods. "No pain, no gain" seems to be the prevailing attitude. The fact is that oncologists pressure their patients to begin receiving chemotherapy immediately. George Crile affirmed in his book, *Cancer and Common Sense* that "those responsible for giving information to the public have chosen to use fear as a weapon. They have created a new disease called cancer phobia, a contagious disease that spreads from mouth to ear."

Just Say No

If surgery, radiation therapy, and chemotherapy have been so unsuccessful, why is it that we have not rejected them? How can this be possible? Is it not our oath to fight, at all costs, for the health and well-being of our patient? According to established decree, there is no other treatment. The only explanation that dismayed scientists have to offer us, after so many years of research and so much money invested and so many lives lost, is that we should continue to use ineffective, dangerous and mutilating methods. Since there is nothing else, they would have us believe that chemotherapy is a necessary evil. Just say NO to tortuous treatment. Natural therapies are effective and improve quality of life unlike chemotherapy and radiation.

When a person turns to a doctor for help, they are giving that physician their trust. Society, until recently, had accepted this state of affairs, trusting in the integrity of the medical professional. Now, the situation is changing. Orthodox physicians are losing the public's trust and this trend worries them. In 1991, the November 4th edition of Time magazine dedicated its cover to "the new era of alternative therapies" and published a report of a survey. In this survey, interviewees were asked first if they had requested help from "alternative doctors" (chiropractors, acupuncturists, herbalists, homeopaths, healers, etc.). Forty-seven percent confessed to having done so. They were also asked if they had considered seeking help from "alternative doctors" in cases where conventional medicine might not have been able to help them. Sixty-two percent answered "YES." The most shocking response was when they were asked: would you go back to the "alternative doctors," Eighty-four percent said "YES!" In other words, they were satisfied with the results alternative therapies gave them. Notice that instead of "quacks," respectfully we are now called "alternative doctors." The survey clearly demonstrates that alternative methods are being sought more frequently. Those methods that the authorities label as "unscientific" are loudly proclaimed by the general public as "more effective." Many would argue that only ignorant people would declare themselves in favor of alternative doctors, but the statistics reveal that a large majority of those interviewed were affluent, university graduates.

Dr. Edward Campion, unremitting critic of alternative methods, published a commentary in the New England Journal of Medicine with the intention of deceiving the reader. He declared that such methods were good for nothing. When he analyzed the phenomenon of the flight of patients to "quackery," he revealed the real problem. The problem, as he saw it, was that "the patients want to feel well." Even as he was speaking ill of alternative medicine, Campion, like a true champion, shot himself in the foot. The public have ceased going to allopathic doctors, who are qualified, specialized, educated, and accredited because these doctors don't make them feel well. Instead, they turn to "quacks" because they make patients feel well again.

In the past, the plagues had the perfect environment in which to spread. Today, even with their serious imperfections, we enjoy urbanized and hygienic cities. To what then are we going to attribute so much illness? As before, we are not taking into consideration the sanitized destruction of the environment -history recycled! Add to that the ineffectiveness of modern health services in general. More and more, the public is pressing the scientific community to seek alternatives to get us out of the dead ends in which we are trapped. The credibility of modern medical science is losing ground fast and the public is gaining information on health matters faster. It seems that the only possible solution is in training ourselves to make responsible choices in the battle for our health.

Menace to Society

The reins of the establishment are tighter on the cancer industry. However, oncologists are not the only ones to care more for their carriers than for their patients. Dr. Philip Caper, an internist and medical policy analyst at Dartmouth Medical School, concludes that the whole medical establishment leaves much to be desired: "I can't imagine a system more dysfunctional than the one we have now — more expensive, not doing the job, with more waste." The General Accounting Office (GAO), estimates that at least 200 billion dollars are thrown away each year on overpriced, useless, even harmful treatments, and on bloated bureaucracy. Every ten years, a group of private researchers for the Rand Company in Santa Monica, California, takes a census of the medical practices in the USA. It reported that a at least 20% of the procedures and treatments offered to patients are not only unnecessary, but life threatening.

Once again, the surgeons are thrust under the spotlight. Cardiovascular surgery is big business. In 1980 about 380,000 cardiac catheterization procedures were done resulting in about 340,000 surgical interventions in the US, according to the Advisory Board Co., a Washington based consulting firm. By 1988 the numbers had swollen, to 965,000 catheterizations and 930,000 interventions. Was all that in the patients' best interest?

Cardiologists are very creative. Hospitals that offer bypass heart surgery are the most lucrative. Dr. Thomas N. James of the University of Texas in Galveston in a report published in the *Journal of the American Medical Association* (JAMA), explained the situation as follows, "The same physician who decides whether a diagnostic procedure is to be done is too often the same one who does the procedure, interprets the findings (and decides whether additional procedures are indicated), and is paid for each step along the way. This is not to say that such physicians are unskillful or that their decisions are necessarily made on the basis of personal gain, but the temptation is inescapably there." In San Diego, California, patients hospitalized for minor heart attacks were reevaluated. Angiograms, that cost between 2000 and 3500 dollars, were prescribed unnecessarily in 40% of the cases. Besides increasing their hospital bills, doctors exposed them to a high risk procedure. Another study, carried out in hospitals in the city of Philadelphia for the implantation of pacemakers, brought to light that 20% were definitively unnecessary and another 36% were implanted "on the basis of

very doubtful criteria." In plain English, not really necessary.

A team of conservative cardiologists in Brigham Hospital,
Boston, evaluated 88 patients that had been scheduled for
cardiac bypass surgery. They advised against surgery for 74
of the 88. Among those 74, 60 accepted a second opinion
and didn't have the operation. These patients were followed
for a period of two years plus. Only two had minor attacks
that could be treated conservatively, an outcome comparable
to that of the 14 (scared not to take the advise of the conservative specialists) patients that underwent open heart surgery. In short, a vast number of patients are submitted to
unnecessary procedures by cardiologists. When surgical
methods for patients with poor heart circulation were popularized in the United States, the death rate of these patients
rose 35% and hospital admissions increased by 50%, according to a study by the University of Arizona. In the United
States, 1 million people die from cardiovascular disease every year. How many people would be alive today if they
had not gone to a cardiologist?

Annually, between 20 million and 25 million surgical procedures are carried out among all the specialties except plastic
surgery. This study determined that between 15% and 29%
were unnecessary. For example, 27% of the women who had
hysterectomies, the second most common surgery, didn't
need the operation! This means that between 3 million and 6
million patients are submitted to surgical risk due to an im-

proper diagnosis or for lucrative reasons. Thank God the anesthesiologists and intensive care specialists have managed to reduce the surgical and post-surgical death rate to 1.33%. This low risk still will not help the over 60,000 that each year have paid with their lives for something they didn't need.

The harm caused by doctors is staggering. Many have denounced the atrocious failures of modern medicine. Adverse reactions to medications recommended by physician account for 659,000 patients hospitalized each year and 16,000 automobile accidents. Over 61,000 people suffer the symptoms of Parkinson's disease induced by pharmaceuticals, but the tragedy of our inefficiency is shamefully exposed by the fact that each year 176,000 people die from drugs prescribed to them by their doctors. This is iatrogenia (death caused by doctor error)! These numbers are drawn from errors recorded in doctors charts. Taking into account the ethical record of the medical business, the findings represent very conservative figures because the charts -probably- had a little "cosmetic surgery" before they were filed. Voltaire showed his wisdom when he insisted that so many fatal errors occur because we prescribe drugs we know little about, in order to treat diseases we know even less about, for patients about whom we know nothing at all. Two hundred years later, Voltaire's conclusion holds firm.

One of the standards imposed by hi-tech American medical practice is diagnostic corroboration through laboratory, x-ray and other invasive tests. I am not in complete disagreement with the criteria but, in my view, they are criminally overused. A very wealthy patient from the border town of Tijuana, Mexico, decided to be treated by a highly trained American doctor in San Diego, California. He returned home in shock because the doctor ordered him to submit to a battery of studies costing more than $2000 dollars before exchanging a single word. When he returned for his evaluative consultation, he indignantly nudged the heap of reports from the doctor's desk and informed him that he had only come for a consultation about an ingrown toenail!

Often doctors who are ill-prepared and doctors who wish to protect themselves against malpractice suits abuse the laboratory and other tests. However, the main reason for the abuse is economic advantage. An investigation by the University of Florida found that a large number of doctors owned laboratories. The investigation showed that such owners require twice the number of tests per patient compared to other doctors. Physicians who have imaging equipment (x-rays, mammography, Tomography, etc.) as part of their offices ordered these studies four times as often as doctors who had to refer their patients to independent x-ray firms. This explains why in the United States there are four times as many MRI's per capita than in Germany where socialized medicine is prevalent.

The Center for Disease Control of the United States reported the following. In the simplest, most routine tests, results were incorrect 30% to 50% of the time. In bacteriological tests where microorganisms were cultured, between 10% and 40% were in error. This can result in the improper prescription of toxic antibiotics. Where results depended on blood samples, between 12% and 15% of the samples were spoiled. Between 12% and 18% of the blood typing tests were inexact. This can cause severe problems for patients in need of blood transfusions. In general, more than 25% of laboratory tests yield unreliable results.

In New Jersey, 225 prestigious laboratories were evaluated. Unknown to these laboratories, several samples from the same patient were sent to different labs. Of the 25,000 tests distributed in this way, only 2 out of 10 were considered highly reliable, while only 5 out of 10 were considered relatively reliable. This means that 30% of the exams were completely untrustworthy. What does this mean? If you take a blood sample from one patient but send several samples with different names to the lab, 30% of the time you are going to get conflicting, erroneous reports. These findings are frightening if you consider that our lives often depend on valid results from laboratory tests.

I have already noted that doctors like to look at the insides of their patients by means of x-ray (especially if the x-ray equipment is their own). You would think that interpreting the images would be a less debatable matter, but the fact is that reading an x-ray film is like reading the Bible. Each person interprets it according to his own point of view. One study reported that 24% of radiologists disagree as to the interpretation of the same x-ray. When they themselves reviewed the same x-ray a second time, 31% of them gave a different diagnosis. Hmm....

In 1955, it was reported that 32% of chest x-rays showing definite abnormalities were erroneously diagnosed as normal. In 1970, a study conducted at the Harvard School of Medicine showed that twenty years later such findings had not improved. When shown a duplicate set of chest x-rays, 56% of the school's radiologists, graduates of the best school of medicine in the world, gave two different diagnoses. Furthermore, in one review of radiographic archives, significant diagnostic errors were detected in 41% of all chest x-rays. In a review of 100 x-rays with colon tumors, 20 studies had been diagnosed as negative, that is to say, the specialists did not see the tumors. As recently as 1994, the *New England Journal of Medicine* informed us that radiologists are mistaken in a "disturbingly high" number of mammogram cases.Due to the popularization of studies without x-ray, like ultra sound and magnetic resonance, x-ray laboratories have changed their designation from x-ray department to *imaging* centers because there they interpret images created by all these apparatuses. I would say that it is because they "imagine" what they interpret. The number of radiological studies is overwhelming. It is calculated that in the United States, 144 million x-rays are done every year. According to studies of those x-rays, 43 million people received treatment for something they didn't have or failed to receive treatment for an existing condition. This is a disturbing situation for a society that is heavily dependent on the doctor. The same results appear with any study that requires interpretation, like electrocardiograms, encephalograms, in fact anything that ends in "-ograms." Think about the following. If, before you boarded a plane, you were told that for every 10 flights 3 planes will crash, would you take the flight? Doctors should rely on the patient's symptoms; not laboratory tests. We must take time to know our patients!

If these atrocities can happen in a country as advanced, regulated, academized, and well-financed as America, what can be expected from those who only imitate without academic or financial support? Experts calculate that the medical faculty of the National University of Mexico (UNAM) is 100 years behind that of Harvard University. If the quality of the doctor truly depended on scholastic pedigree and resources, imagine what the iatrogenic death rate in Mexico or other less affluent countries would be. American medical services are the most expensive. In fact, 80% of the bankruptcies reported are due to medical expenses.

Of the 24 industrialized countries belonging to the Organization of Economic Corporation and Development (OED), the United States -even though it spends more than twice the money on health care than **all** the other members combined they barely made number 20! Dr. Barbara

Starfield of the School of Public Health at Johns Hopkins, compares the state of health of her fellow countrymen with nine industrialized European countries and the United States was classified in last place. Maybe the Harvard medical students should save a lot of money and go to school in Mexico.

Sometimes I ask myself why do the doctors, Mexican and from all over the world, want to emulate the dehumanized American school of medicine? I don't deny that the economic situation and general underdevelopment of our country deprives the Mexican physician of many luxuries. Yet, it is clear that the answer does not lie in excess. Nor does being an economic power guarantee better medical attention. We (and all countries) should maintain a medical identity in line with our resources and cultural values. Medicine is more art than science.

In 1993, the National Academy of Medicine in Mexico evaluated medical services in the United States, Canada and Mexico in preparation for NAFTA. The most important factors studied were infant mortality, average life span and cost of services. No one was surprised that Mexico had the most deficient services, but it was definitively surprising that health indexes were better in Canada than in the United States. Mexico has 130 doctors for every 100,000 inhabitants and had the worst infant mortality rate and the lowest average life span. The United States, 586 doctors per 100,000 inhabitants, spends ten times more than the

Canadians and 100 times more than the Mexicans in health care. Could it be that Canada, to reach the best rate of the three countries had more than, say... 700 doctors per 100,000? No, in fact, for every 100,000 Canadians there are only 57 physicians. Surprised? Maybe you shouldn't be.

The German health authorities designed a study to prove that pollution and stress play an important role in death rates. They wanted to scientifically determine why people living in rural areas live longer and better than those living in more populated areas. The gun backfired on them. The most important factor turned out to be neither stress nor pollution; instead it was the fact that rural areas had less doctors per capita. Translation? The more doctors there are around you, the higher the death rate!

History confirms the findings of the German investigation and the NAFTA study. In fact, in all cases where doctors went on strike, the death rate dropped significantly. This phenomenon appeared on several occasions. During 1973 in Israel, doctors went on strike reducing the daily consultation load from 65,000 to 7,000. The strike lasted one month and, surprisingly, the death rate dropped by 50%. In 1976, in Bogota, Colombia, doctors attended only emergency cases during a 52 day strike. The death rate was reduced by 35%. The same reduction (35%) in the death rate happened in Brazil when medical services were suspended for almost two months. Also in 1976, the death rate was reduced by 18% in a strike in Los Angeles, California, and operations dropped by 60%. When doctors suspended the strike, the death rates soared above and beyond the rates prevailing before the strike. It would seem that doctors returned to work with renewed vigor. Doctors… morticians best friends. Unbelievable!

When medical authorities were questioned as to their opinion regarding the collapse of the death rate during the strikes, the experts explained that "during the strikes they attend only emergencies and were not distracted, all their energy was concentrated to attending those who were truly sick." It gives me true pleasure to point out a conclusion from a physician that actually makes sense, but why is it then hat doctors have not declared a perpetual strike?

Alternative Medicine

By 1994, everyone was talking about alternative therapies. The magazine *MPLS St. Paul* dedicated its cover to acupuncture, herbalism, therapeutic massage, macrobiotic diet, chiropractic and others in an article entitled "New Ways of Healing" in which it was reported that even orthodox hospitals were allowing the admission of alternative services, not because they believe in them but to recuperate lost clientele. The issue that broke all sales records for *Time* magazine appeared on April 6, 1995. The cover displayed a variety of vitamin tablets and capsules and bore the title "The Power of Vitamins. New research shows they may help in the war against cancer, cardiac disease and the ravages of aging."

In the face of the atrocious results of orthodox cancer treatments, the public has decided to look to those alternatives criticized by the establishment. They are moving toward answers that are rejected by those who continue to waste their time in laboratories. Government authorities and scientists, in spite of the overwhelming quantity of studies from the world's universities, want to keep us tied to the belief that there is nothing apart from the approved treatments, and that the proposed alternative therapies lack scientific bases. Beyond all doubt, Heinrich Himmler, Hitler's director of propaganda, was right when he said that if a lie is repeated often enough, people will accept it as the truth. If the authorities were impartial, they would prohibit the approved treatments for cancer since scientifically, they have been demonstrated to be useless. Beyond that, clinical studies have demonstrated that these treatments endanger the quality of life and are often deadly.

Who Are The Real Quacks?

The authorities gravely censure alternative therapies for a variety of reasons. Dr. Casseleth, Advisor to the Office for Alternative Therapies, a recently created government office, which evaluates such therapies, summarizes their main objections as follows: "While it is well to keep an open mind, it is wise to keep one's eyes open also. Many alternative therapies are not risky, except to our pocketbooks, but some can be dangerous. Do not substitute an alternative therapy for treatment already accepted." Here are some of

the accusations levied against alternative medicine by
Casseleth followed by my response to each:

Casseleth's Accusations

1. They promise miraculous healing and offer false hope.
2. They involve secret procedures or ingredients.
3. Therapies aren't allowed to reach the public due to some
   conspiracy.
4. They involve exorbitant cost.
5. They report exaggerated positive results backed only by
   anecdotal case histories.
6. They invite us to abandon or delay proven medical
   treament.

My Responses

1. I agree that if someone says that he is able to cure every dis
   ease, he has a God complex and is dangerous. Yet, supporters
   of orthodox medicine sin even more when they prohibit alternatives for problems for which they have nothing to offer.
   They assert that if orthodox medicine has not found a solution, no one can find it. A false hope is one which has neither
   scientific basis nor proven results. Do they possess a true
   hope? Do they have scientifically proven treatments? No.
   What they really offer is a quick death. "Go home and settle
   your affairs because you are going to die in a few months.

Don't waste money on alternative therapies," they say.
So much for hope.

2.   The criticism of secrecy seems very strange to me, since
the foundation of modern medicine is cemented with patents that protect the secrecy of drugs. But when a medical "quack" discovers a method that guarantees longevity,
it is judged as secretive. I will admit, however, that I believe creative methodology which helps the sick should
be shared.

3.   I counter Casseleth's cries of conspiracy with a question.
What do you call an establishment which protects its market and investments by criticizing alternative therapies
and abusing laws and rules to suppress their chance for
survival? Don't call it conspiracy, call it what it really is
- the establishment.

4.   On the issue of cost Dr. Casseleth really bit her tongue.
According to *the New England Journal of Medicine*
(1994), alternative therapies are sixty times cheaper than
conventional ones. I have already mentioned that 82% of
the patients who consulted the so called "quacks" were
satisfied with the treatment received. Who has to be satisfied, the authorities or the patients? The cost of orthodox oncological treatments is truly exorbitant.

5.   In comparison to orthodox therapies for chronic degenerative diseases, the results of alternative therapies are un-
believably superior. Yet, even though they are backed by

a multitude of studies, as we saw in the case of breast cancer, they are omitted, ignored, or they are impossible to carry out.

6. In other words, alternative therapies may pose a serious threat when a patient, if swayed toward alternatives, loses the opportunity to receive the (extremely) effective orthodox treatment? Run that by me again! Time and time again it has been confirmed that the "proven medical treatments" are not only ineffective but dangerous. The vast majority of patients with cancer live longer and better if left without the orthodox treatments. Oncologists will not accept these treatments for themselves. No scientific research is needed to prove that fresh vegetables, fruit, juices, medicinal herbs, vitamins, minerals, fiber, etc. are not harmful to the body. It would be nice if there were proof that surgery, radiation, and chemotherapy were not harmful.

In short, people like Dr. Casseleth may criticize alternative doctors and treatments galore, but the fact is that more and more doctors are becoming interested in alternative therapies. Associations like the American College of Advanced Medicine (ACAM), and other associations are quickly jumping on the bandwagon. Hundreds of doctors are recommending or using alternative therapies in their offices, almost all, according to Dr. Bruckheim from Tribune Media Services, are satisfied with the results and are going to continue prescribing them.

Hospitals

The failure of the medical community does not end with the doctors. It has invaded their sacred workplace, the shiny anti-septic hospitals. A story that made the front page of the Boston *Globe* in March of '95 shook the USA. Betsy Lehman, a health columnist for this prestigious newspaper since 1982, died at the Dana-Farber Cancer Institute, a world renown hospital affiliated with Harvard Medical School. The cause was a huge overdose of chemotherapy administered by the hospital's staff. "Three large studies over the last 30 years have documented a distressingly consistent rate of medical mishaps in the US" Christine Gorman of Time magazine reported in April of '95, "Lehman's case is just one of a spate of medical foul-ups that have made the headlines in recent weeks." The wrong leg of a patient was amputated and the hospital ended up amputating the other later. A radical mastectomy done on a Michigan woman claimed the breast without the cancer, then the diseased one had to be removed. A four year old girl, hours after a tonsillectomy, died at home from a massive hemorrhage.

Are these isolated cases? "Just in the state of New York, poor medical attention was translated into the death of 7,000 patients in a single year, according to investigators from the Harvard Medical School. Extrapolated on a national level, this discovery suggests that deficient medical attention may be linked to some 80,000 deaths every year," reports Walt Bogdanich, in his book entitled *The Great White Lie*.

Authors Inlander, Levine and Weiner, in their book *Medicine on Trial*, also criticize aspects of the medical community in the United States. They criticize the corruption in hospitals and detail the repercussions on patients. They claim that hospitals illegally reuse disposable devices to cut costs. Many of these devices have been designed to use one time, but are only washed before being used again to reduce costs. But the perpetrators are careful to cover their tracks, because if the patient knew about the substitution, they would have legal grounds for a lawsuit. In one hospital survey, employees reported routinely reusing disposable catheters and their guides, respiratory circuits and biopsy needles. Another survey rendered even more frightening information. Interviewees reported reusing high risk materials like manual resuscitators, orthopedic prostheses, anesthesia masks, and so on. According to Allen L. Otten of the Wall Street Journal, one hospital admitted having reused some catheters up to 45 times.

Some disposable materials are constructed well enough to be reused with a low margin of risk. This practice might be acceptable or even commendable in a hospital in a poverty ridden country. But it seems criminal that such a practice should be carried out in private hospitals, where patients pay elevated prices, and assume that everything is being done to reduce the risk of acquiring contagious diseases. What makes the problem of reuse even worse is that often untrained people "recondition" these disposable items, increasing the risk of danger for the patient.

There are many factors that contribute to poor medical attention. Unfortunately people often die from such shoddy practices. Bogdanich points out that, "In 1988, doctors serving the federal government made a scandalizing discovery in Parsons Hospital in Queens, New York. More than half the patients who died in a six month period were victims of the negligence of the hospital staff. In spite of that, there were no legal reprisals or legal repercussions because families of the deceased were not informed of the cause of death. The hospital was simply closed and the employees were quietly transferred to other institutions within the city."

In the United States, hospitals are obliged to take in poor patients with the understanding that they will be later reimbursed for such services by the government through a program called "Medicare." If these people are turned away, institutions may be subjected to heavy sanctions. This is a service which the United States government provides to its poor and underprivileged. Yet, in a 1991 survey, it was reported that 140 American hospitals routinely reject patients who generate no income in spite of the fact that it is absolutely illegal for them to do so. Sanctions were imposed on only 19 of the hospitals, an open invitation to other hospitals to take the risk. Even when a certain number of indigents were admitted to a hospital, a study at the national level revealed that the death rate among the poor was triple that of insured patients. Am I contradicting myself? Does the health establishment really work? I doubt it, when such people go to the hospital it is obviously for a critical emergency -where medicine really shines- but if at the same time an insured person, and potentially sue-happy, has come in with a tooth ache, the non-paying patient will not receive attention. This is the real reason why there will be more fatalities among poor patients than among the affluent.

Law suits against doctors and hospitals are commonplace in the United States. Many plaintiffs have received truly staggering settlements. In spite of this, such legal actions have not improved the medical profession. They have only served to make it more inaccessible. Patients have to undergo all sorts of unnecessary tests so that doctors can generate enough money to protect themselves from the possibility of malpractice. The answer is not to sue but to change the system.

In spite of deficient medical attention, hospitals charge exorbitant amounts for their services. On the TV program "Prime Time," on January 12, 1995, Diane Sawyer reported that an accident victim was transported to the hospital by helicopter and spent only five hours there before expiring. His relatives were forced to pay more than 94,000 dollars in hospital expenses and more than 10,000 dollars for doctors' honorariums. There was no doubt that the boy was treated with the sincere desire to save his life but $104,000 dollars for just five hours? Even for rich Americans, this is ridiculous.

One of the strongest and best founded fears of patients regarding hospitals is the food. They are shocked by their lack of seasoning, but the problem goes far beyond that. It is logical to think that in the case of illness or accidents, nutritional requirements must necessarily be taken into account. Udeniably, adequate nutrition is inseparably linked to health. Disease increases in direct proportion to malnutrition, thus properly nourished patients have more resources for combating disease. The deficient nutritional value of hospital food prolongs illness and therefore the length of the hospital stay. It would seem that doctors, nutritionists and dietitians along with administrators, have not been able to understand this simple but vital natural law of nutrition since the diet offered to patients while hospitalized is deprived of nutrients. Or, do you suppose that besides saving money in cheap food they hope to increase revenues by prolonging the hospital stay? This is what we call killing two birds with one stone. Lamentably, it is not birds that get killed. The consequences are awful. According to a report in *Forbes* magazine, 50,000 hospital deaths each year are directly related to the food served to the patients while hospitalized.

The word hospital comes from Latin, "hospitalis" which means hospitable, generous, and beneficent. However, many hospitals are no longer inviting, no longer treating people in a caring, amiable way. A hospital's atmosphere plays a vital role in the pursuit of health. Our Oasis of Hope Hospital has been decorated in mauve, warm colors with more of a four star hotel setting. Pleasant settings not only make the patients feel well, it has been proven in studies that patients who are housed in a pleasant environment, who are made to feel in control of the situation, and who get answers to their questions respond better to treatment. It is a disgrace that our bright white and shiny hospitals are so inhospitable, cold and sterile in their treatment of patients.

So it is, in the course of history, that we have gone through the fear of the unknown, to the fear of germs but, in spite of the valiant warfare and development of unbelievable medical weaponry, the germs seem to be up on the scoreboard. The world continues to face many of the same and some new plagues. That's the way life is. What is unacceptable is that we, the doctors, have become a menace to society.

I have kept you in the dark long enough about the title of this chapter, but after all this information, it's easier to explain the Mexican saying that inspired it. If you have read the Bible, you know that the number of the beast is 666. In Mexico, the number 111 is given to doctors. Why 111? Because doctors believe that life begins with one (the doctor's birthing expertise), it continues with one (doctors care throughout the life), and it [he] *finishes* with one (especially if "euthankevorkianasia"…or whatever, is your doctor's spacialty!).

Doctors have to change their professional philosophy and motivation. Prestige and profit rule medical practice. Abuses of diagnostic and treatment procedures have driven costs in money and lives through the roof. Less interventionism is one of the answers. How many centuries did we survive without cardiologists, surgeons and gynecologists? Was our race at any time threatened for lack of them? I do believe that doctors have a place in society, but their intervention must be guided by a different set of rules if the medical race wants to survive in the 21st century.

Chapter 5

The Possible Dream

They are giants and if you are afraid, don't get in my way and
start praying in the meantime I'm going to engage
them in fierce and unequal battle.

Don Quixote

Don Quixote, The Man Of La Mancha, began a crusade
across Spain to fight for the triumph of good, justice, beauty
and love. In the previous quote, the honorable Don
Quixote was admonishing his servant, Sancho, for trying to
convince lord Quixote that the "enemies" before him were

not giants, they were only windmills! Miguel de Cervantes y Saavedra, the Spanish author of this masterpiece, demonstrates through this beautiful novel, that in order to reach the unreachable, **madness** is a prerequisite.

False Philosophy

Today, the condition of the medical profession is demoralizing, to say the least. We must examine the reasons for such failure. Yes, modern technology is inviting, our colleagues are instrumental and the authorities are more that persuasive to keep us in the arena of the establishment's medical industry. When the "establishment's blindfolds" of a doctor occasionally come down, the gigantic errors (horrors) of the medical industry come into full view, but the "big brothers" of the establishment tell us that we are just looking at windmills. Are science and technology truly to blame? Are the authorities forcing doctors to practice mechanized medicine? No, doctors have the choice between the establishment and the patients. The rewards of the establishment are prestige and money; the consequences I've outlined in chapter 4. The rewards of true, artful medicine are satisfied, happy patients; the doctors' consequences, ostracism and disgrace. It all comes down to a moral and philosophical compromise.

In the United States, against all medical principles and moral values (now outdated), abortion was legalized. The original Hippocratic Oath clearly proscribed abortion, this part was conveniently changed to "...will give no drug, perform no operation, *for criminal purpose...*" Because abortions are now performed under the law, there is no criminal purpose. American doctors perform more than one million annually. In America today, the most unsafe place for a baby is the mother's womb. I know a nurse who, at the age of 54, decided to quit her job at a hospital because they performed abortions there. She knew that at 54 getting another job would be difficult, but her principles took precedence over her monetary needs. Courage like hers is a rarity today.

Most of what used to matter doesn't any more. Today's generation lives by a very different sort of values. Our moral foundation has changed. James Patterson and Peter Kim in their book *The Day America Told The Truth*, concluded that the modern ten commandments that Americans live by are:

I.   There is no reason to observe the day of rest (I don't believe in God).

II.   I will steal from those who won't really miss it.

III.   I will lie when it suits me, so long as it doesn't cause any real damage.

IV.   I will drink and drive if I feel I can handle it. I know my limit.

V.   I will cheat on my spouse. After all, given the chance, he or she will do the same.

VI.   I will procrastinate at work and do absolutely nothing about one full day in every five. It's standard operating procedure.

VII.   I will use recreational drugs.

VIII.   I will cheat on my taxes - to a point.

IX.   I will put my lover at risk of disease, I sleep around a bit, but who doesn't?

X.   Technically, I may have committed date rape, but I know that she wanted it.

Eroding traditional values are not limited to Americans; the moral fabric of today's world societies leave much to be desired and certainly doctors are not the exception. Modern medical practices have broken the most rudimentary principles of medicine. The first was established by Hippocrates more than 2,500 years ago, *"Primum Est Nil Nocere"* (First, and Foremost, Do No Harm) The second principle also was established almost twenty centuries ago by Jesus Christ when He said, "Love your neighbor as you love yourself." Translated into the medical profession this statement would read, "Love your patients as you love yourself."

Unfortunately, many of the treatments doctors recommend to their patients, are treatments they themselves would elect not to receive. For example, the colonoscopic examination is a commonly recommended exam. In it a hose more than a yard long with a diameter of a human thumb is introduced into the rectum. Those of us that have personally experienced this embarrassing and uncomfortable procedure surely hesitate before recommending it. I'm not saying this study is worthless but definitively overused, in most cases because the payment for the colonoscope is due.

The options modern mechanized physicians have now are limitless, it seems. Tests, procedures, interventions and treatments are accessible weapons used in the "patient's interest," without restriction. It is public knowledge that doctors make the worst patients. People think this is because we are stubborn and in a hurry. In reality, doctors are reluctant patients because we have insider information and are well aware of the risks of medical intervention. Fear is quicker than lighting! The day that physicians love their patients as themselves, their armamentarium will suddenly shrink to what they are willing to take themselves.

Outcasts are the doctors that practice such retrograde medicine. Not to take "advantage" of modernization is heresy and will not be tolerated! Few are willing to suffer criticism, pressure and even persecution for the principles to which we pledged. Instead, we are tied to the status quo, the medical machinery and its earnings. My father, Dr. Ernesto Contreras Sr., who has been a powerful influence in my life, as in the lives of a host of health professionals who today are offering alternative therapies to their patients around the globe, is one of those courageous outcasts.

Medicine's Man From La Mancha

When I was 12 years old, because of an illness that kept me in bed for a few days, my mother gave me the book of the "Man From La Mancha" the story of <u>Don</u> <u>Quixote,</u> bound in two enormous volumes, to help wile away the hours. When I saw the size of the books, I decided I would only look at the illustrations but I soon found myself taken up in the story's content. I enjoyed reading already but The <u>Quixote</u> was the first book to ever completely take away my desire for sleep. I devoured it night and day down to the last page. Joe Darion, author of the lyrics for "The Impossible Dream," depicted the story of this madman with an incredible vision, powerful enough to change the world. The concept of dreaming the impossible, fighting the unbeatable and reaching the unreachable, had a profound influence in my life until even today my closest friends criticize me as an unredeemable dreamer and optimist. A long time passed before I realized I was living under the same roof with a man of La Mancha, a Don Quixote. Even down to the lack of hair and lanky build, my father resembles that good gentleman and, like Don Quixote, he wasn't just another lunatic as most of his friends and colleagues thought. He was simply a man captivated by the madness of an unreachable goal, the triumph over the hopelessness of the sick. He armed himself with "quixotesque" antiquated and bygone weaponry of the true medicine, refusing to embrace the tools of the modern physician. Today's cold professional has forgotten the art of healing. My father has fought all of his life for the triumph of good, justice, beauty, and love of medicine and his patients. These are values doctors have lost in the exercise of their profession. The taunts and humiliations along the way did not stop him in his quest to reach the unreachable star.

In the 1960s, my father was one of the most promising doctors in the field of oncology. He was one of the founders of the Oncological Society and Pathological Society in Mexico. He specialized at Harvard University in pediatric clinical pathology and was, at that time, a very well known and recognized orthodox physician. However, in 1966, as he explains in his autobiography *To You, My Beloved Patient*, his life changed radically after traveling around the world with my mother, my oldest sister and her husband. They visited Pergamum, an ancient Greek city of northwest Asia Minor, in Mysia (now Turkey) where once a group of scholars established a school of grammatical study in opposition to the scholars of the Alexandrian library. Under Roman control, Pergamum remained one of the chief cities of Asia Minor and the capital of the province of Asia. The ruins of the ancient city surround the modern town of Bergama. Noted for its splendor, the city's ruins include a Roman theater, an amphitheater, and a circus.

A guide, knowing that my father was a doctor, decided to take him on an extended tour of the ruins. He showed my father an ancient sanitarium. It was very different from the hospitals we now know because the patients had to pass through three buildings. In the first building, patients met with religious counselors. They believed in the need to be evaluated spiritually. In the second building, patients met with a psychologist of sorts who evaluated their mental state. In the last building, they received a physical evaluation. The concept shook my father. The hospital in Pergamum was a place for healing the whole man, not just his body. After Pergamum, my father was enlightened by this vision. It was a light he had to follow.

In those days, my father practiced the "exact" science of medicine, making diagnoses with the help of the microscope. After his voyage, he felt a tremendous burden. His work sentenced patients he didn't even know, to death. Even worse he had to explain that the available treatments promised suffering but not healing. He began to focus more on the patient than on the patient's tissue samples. He didn't keep this discovery to himself, but began to divulge it to his colleagues in the medical society. He wanted to discuss the idea of loving the patient, taking into account spiritual and emotional needs. He reminded his colleagues of the atrocities effected by surgery, radiation and chemotherapy, and encouraged them to seek less aggressive, more natural and less toxic therapies. The response of his peers was immediate. Applause? No, he was promptly expelled from the medical establishment and professionally exiled. The man had gone mad. It was the year of our Lord, 1967.

This blow was exactly what the divine physician had prescribed for him. Though his enemies were true giants, he did not throw his hands up in despair but, like Don Quixote, said, "I am going to engage them in fierce and unequal battle." He began to carry out what he considered to be his mission, in spite of the severe harsh criticism of his colleagues. Already excommunicated from the medical guild, he became a pioneer in the practice of holistic medicine and alternative therapies. He promoted the idea that orthodox therapies should be applied in a less aggressive form. He preached that proper diet and detoxification were equal or superior to any therapeutic method, alternative or orthodox. He instituted programs to help patients with their emotional problems. He studied the causes of stress and sought ways to enrich the spirit of his patients. As a result, the success of our hospital has been better than that of the famous oncological centers around the world. Dreaming the impossible is the only way to make things possible.

When our manner of treatment has been evaluated by other scientists, they attempt to minimize our success by insinuating that our patients were misdiagnosed. They often claim that the patients didn't even have cancer. Sometimes they assert that the treatments we offer didn't help the patient, but the patient merely experienced "spontaneous remission." In fact, they will probably never give my father the recognition he deserves. However, if he is entered in the book of records, he will be registered as "the healer with the patients who experienced the highest rate of spontaneous remission in the history of medicine."

I deeply admire my father for his intelligence, knowledge, and enormous clinical ability, as well as his "touch" with patients because after spending only a few minutes with him, they already feel relief. But what I will admire even more for the rest of my life is that he made whatever sacrifice necessary so that his patients had access to "alternatives" when the "accepted" treatments were so clearly ineffective. He wasn't intimidated when he lost his position as a renowned scientist, or when he was challenged by establishment oncologists, or when authorities closed him down, or when money was tight. He didn't even shrink from the worst, that his prestige be tainted with mud from the swamps of quackery. He faced all this persecution harboring in his heart the "call" to attend the needs of his patients and of his patients only. Thanks to his efforts, less aggressive and more natural treatments are available to many.

I feel proud when I see other clinics, hospitals and private physicians embrace these concepts, once so firmly ridiculed. According to Dr. Bruckheim (*Tribune Media Services*), a survey pointed out that 30% of all doctors frequently steer their patients to alternative therapies, 74% admitted to having used unconventional remedies in their consultation rooms, and 67% have occasionally sought the help of alternative doctors for their patients. Of those brave souls who have personally experimented with unorthodox methods, 91% say they would do so again. In the MD Anderson Hospital, they now practice conservative surgery for breast cancer. My father promoted this kind of surgery 30 years ago and was called a quack. The Mayo Clinic recently published a book on the power of nutrition, but 30 years ago it ridiculed my father for affirming that diet played an important role in the prevention and treatment of cancer. First they ridiculed his hypotheses, then they fought them "scientifically", and now they have appropriated them as their own. Walking shoulder to shoulder, as son and disciple with a "Quixote" for the ideal practice of medicine that is truly art-science, full of love and hope for patients, is and will be the greatest privilege that God has given me. His loving madness empowered him to reach what everybody thought was unreachable.

Philosophy of the Contreras Care Center at The Oasis of Hope Hospital

The unique nature of our institution does not lie in the impressiveness of our building nor in the modern equipment we have. It does not lie in the diplomas our doctors have acquired from universities or even from the nature of the treatment we give. What sets our hospital apart from the other oncological centers of the world is the fact that we give unprecedented attention to the close relationship that exists between the disease and its host. This would seem to be logical, but it is the least common approach in modern medicine.

Today's doctors are obsessed with diseases so much so that they know nothing about health. If an apparently healthy patient comes to us, we either make him ill or we allow him to continue with habits that sicken him. It is no secret that the most costly failure of medicine in the 20th century is the treatment of cancer. Surgery, radiation, and chemotherapy not only fail to help patients, but often destroy their quality of life. The inadequacy of these therapies is that they focus only on the tumor. The host is cast aside. It doesn't even matter whether the patient suffers. If the patient gets worse, he is often criticized for failing to respond correctly to the therapy. In other words, the patient is at fault. How convenient, patients die on us because they don't know how to respond!

In our hospital, our principal focus is the patient. The treatments are designed to improve the quality of the patient's life. What separates us from the rest is our philosophy. Our mission is based on the two fundamental principles of medicine: do no harm and love thy patient as thyself. The anticancer therapies of the present establishment have brutally broken these universal medical principles. Orthodox treatments severely injure patients and oncologists rarely prescribe these treatments for their loved ones, much less for themselves.

In our hospital, we involve the patient in the treatment decision-making process. We never use therapies that deteriorate the patient's quality of life. We provide them with treatments that improve the quality of their lives. Sometimes we use an orthodox treatment if it is absolutely necessary and will improve the patient's health. For example, if a patient's tumor is blocking the digestive tract, natural therapies would be inadequate because they take a long time to reduce tumor size. The patient's life is threatened in a mater of hours, at most-days; surgery not only significantly improves the quality of his life, it saves the patient. In the same way, there are other examples where chemotherapy and radiation therapy may be helpful; we know the tumor reduction is not permanent, but it gives us the time needed for the alternative therapy to work. The problem is not in the therapies themselves but in the criteria which govern their application.

Yet, patients need a treatment that will attack the root of the problem. Natural therapies destroy tumors slowly through internal mechanisms (immunities). These nontoxic therapies give the body the weapons it needs to fight illness. They are not symptomatic therapies but they truly attack the foundation of illness. My father established the criteria that gave birth to these alternative treatments in Mexico.

Other clinics and hospitals have "anti-tumor" programs which are rigid and inflexible, like a shoe shop which only offers one size; the consumer must fit into the shoe! The mission of our oncologists is to find an adequate treatment specific to the needs of each patient. We are eclectic in our approach. In over 30 years, we've had the opportunity to evaluate many products and alternative remedies, like shark cartilage, cat's claw, herbs, homeopathic products, nontoxic medicines, electro-magnetic fields, etc. We research all avenues that seem promising, have sufficient scientific basis, suggest efficacy, and are nontoxic. But everything must fit into our philosophy. The treatment must not negatively affect the quality of the patient's life and we must use treatments we would choose for ourselves if the need arose. The medical industry, seemingly with limitless treatment options, suddenly has very little to offer that meets those simple requirements, but God has provided everything we need for our health maintenance in nature. The most natural and least aggressive modalities are offered. We improve the patient's ability to fight disease by providing the body, mind, and soul with the tools they need. In other words, we are not in the business of getting rid of tumors (nor patients). God gave us the capacity to heal ourselves, our mission is to provide the necessary resources for our patients to get well.

Metabolic Therapy

Originally, my father called it "holistic therapy" because he recognized that, to obtain the best results, one had to treat the patient in the physical, emotional, and spiritual spheres. The term "holistic" has been adopted by many followers; among them, "New Age" therapists with humanistic or anti-Christian religious philosophy. In order to not be confused with persons that profess these philosophies, we now use the term "Metabolic Therapy." Metabolism is the total function of our body and so that it can be carried out efficiently, all its attributes should work in harmony: body, mind and spirit. Caring for our patients in *totality* is the goal of the **metabolic therapy**. This goal is achieved through several branches: Detoxification, Diet, Immune Stimulation and Anti-Tumor Agents; each with the objective of providing resources to create the best environment in our organism to fight while at the same time making the cancer cells unwelcome.

Detoxification

Once again I insist that our health, and lastly our lives, depend basically on two things: the intake of the necessary nutrients and the output of waste. The fact that there are more organs designated for the latter should indicate the importance of detoxification. Many of the toxins found in the air, ground, water, food and medicines remain in our bodies causing serious damage. At times, these poisons permanently imbed themselves in our tissues. Our bodies are often so besieged by toxins, that the organs designed for elimination of waste (colon, liver, kidneys, lungs and skin) are overwhelmed and incapacitated. Therefore, an integral part of metabolic therapy is detoxification. We have developed methods that can effectively help the body get rid of these toxins. High fiber preparations increase intestinal passage. Colonics and enemas helpclean the lower intestinal tract. Intravenous solutions with amino acids (EDTA) pick up toxic substances and eliminate them in the urine.

Breathing exercises, and oxygen therapy are also intregral parts in the detoxification process. Finally, there are natural substances that increase hepatic detoxification like milk thistle, garlic, etc. Used in conjunction with each other, the body is assisted in the task of eliminating harmful toxins that block the normal function, a "clean" body is in better shape for battle.

Diet

We cannot avoid the ravages of the environment but, in great measure, we control the food we put in our mouths. While in the hospital, our patients consume natural organically grown foods without preservatives or toxins. Whole grain cereals and breads. Foods loaded with nutrients like vitamins, phytochemicals, flavonoids, minerals, proteins, and fiber.

In the 20s, the Nobel Prize for medicine was awarded to Dr. Otto Warburg for discovering that malignant cells obtain their energy mainly from proteins and fats, while normal cells produce their energy almost exclusively from carbohydrates. Few indeed are those who make use of this vital information. Based on these scientific facts, my father initiated the use of food as an anti-cancer therapy more than 30 years ago, recommending that his patients ingest a diet rich in complex carbohydrates (fruits and vegetables), poor in protein and very low in fat (fatty meats and milk products). God's plan is that we eat things which provide enough nutrients to prevent disease and to maintain health.

Sadly enough, modern scientists and physicians have largely disregarded such natural laws.

Immune Stimulation

The relevance of the immune system, the organization that protects our bodies from aggressors, has been underestimated since Pasteur, but the tragedy of AIDS has brought it forward. The resolution of any disease depends ultimately on the integrity of this system of defense. Cancer is called an opportunistic disease because it takes advantage of the body's inability to defend itself from tumors developing and invading it. In reality all diseases are opportunistic. Our immune system is now too often forced to work overtime against an environment filled with destructive and carcinogenic agents.

The foods we eat are depleted of nutrients, cheating the immune system of much needed resources. We are not going to leave nutrient intake to chance. Mega-doses of vitamins, minerals, phytochemicals and amino acids are administered to our patients continuously. In addition, we live in a society that places tremendous physical, emotional and spiritual demands on us, creating a destructive level of stress. Scientific research reports that this stress severely depresses the immune system. Stress reducing techniques are very important. Therefore, as part of the immune stimulation program, we offer patients psychological and spiritual counseling. Through them, all patients have the option of participating in spiritual programs where they have the opportunity to have a personal encounter with God. The separation of medicine and faith is another flagrant flaw of the modern science of medicine. I will amplify these concepts but suffice it to say for now that it's a pity doctors don't turn to the Almighty for assistance more often. With a clean and immune stimulated patient, the weapons aimed at the tumor directly are much more effective.

Anti-Tumor Agents

Cancer has no word of honor. Those who say that it's easy to treat have enlightenment we don't or are the ultimate in naïveté. We must use all resources at hand to combat this incredibly stubborn and effective enemy. Remember that our goal is not to destroy tumors, but to provide quality of life. Nature provides no small arsenal to destroy tumors or at least to neutralize their growth. Natural cancer-busters like shark cartilage, garlic, vitamin A, urea, selenium, etc. are at our disposition, but we have at arms length whatever will improve the quality of life of our patients.

The branch of the therapy that focuses an attack on the tumors is founded on the use of *Amygdalin*, better known as "Laetrile." This natural, anti-tumor agent has been the source of many conflicts. I'm not going to abound in this theme, material of many books, but concentrate on explaining the reason for its efficacy. Chemically speaking, Laetrile is a diglucoside (a sugar) with a cyanide radical. It exists in all seeds, except citrus, and in many plants. It has been used by Egyptian doctors for curative purposes since the time of the Pharaohs and it was already recorded to be in use in the year 2800 B.C. by a Chinese herbalist (Pen Tsao). It is a successful but maligned alternative cancer treatment. Researchers began studying the substance because the Hunza tribes in the Himalayas enjoy one of the lowest incidence of cancer in the world. Their main source of protein is apricot kernels, one of the best sources of Amygdalin.

The Pueblo Indians of Taos, New Mexico, traditionally eat many foods rich in Amygdalin. Not coincidentally, cancer is rare among this population. Robert G. Houston, who has written several articles on the Pueblo, was given a recipe by them as he researched for a book on cancer prevention: In a glass of milk or juice, mix a tablespoon of honey with a quarter ounce, or two dozen, freshly ground apricot kernels; or one kernel for every ten pounds of body weight. Houston wrote that the drink was so delicious he had it daily.

Dr. Ernest Krebs Jr. found that Amygdalin was protecting these people from developing cancer and called it vitamin B17. Later, his research group found that Amygdalin also had powerful cancer killer capabilities because it contains cyanide that destroys cancer cells. Already judged as therapeutically ineffective, health officials now claimed that laetrile was also a poison! Interestingly, we constantly eat produce with cyanide, about 1200 natural foods have it. We have treated over 40,000 patients with high dosages of

Amygdalin and never had one case of cyanide poisoning. Krebs found enzymes that activate (beta-glucosidase) and neutralize (rhodenase) cyanide in our bodies. Cancer cells have a 3600 fold concentration of beta-glucosidase and are extremely deficient in rhodenase. That is why naturally occurring cyanide is so devastating for malignant tumors. Rhodenase, the cyanide neutralizing enzyme, is very abundant in our bodies and detoxifies the cyanide released by foods and Laetrile. It's God's way. Samuel Waksman, a famous pharmacology expert said, "The cures for all man's diseases already exist in the world around us. It is the task of science to recognize them." Amygdalin is a natural chemotherapy, effective and completely nontoxic. Furthermore, when the Amygdalin breaks down it produces a very strong pain killer, another blessing for patients with tumors. Amygdalin is extraordinarily effective in common tumors like carcinomas of the prostate, breast, colon and lungs, as well as lymphomas. Twenty years ago, German scientists reported that proteolytic enzymes could aid Amygdalin by synergism. Since then both are given together, resulting in an improvement of our statistics.

In spite of scientific and clinical reports about the efficacy of Laetrile in the treatment of cancer, the health authorities such as the California State Department of Public Health said that patients taking it were literally taking their life in their own hands! Jay Hutchinson, a Laetrile activist wrote the following mock letter to the King of Hunzaland to accentuate the stupidity of the situation (I will paraphrase):

I'm rushing this extremely urgent warning to you so that you can take immediate steps to notify your government and your people of the health hazard reported by the California State Department of Public Health during the week of September 3, 1972.

....it is a time for action. King, you must get your people to stop eating those [apricot] pits! Stop making flour out of them! Stop feeding your newborn infants the oil, and for Mohammed's sake, stop anointing them with it!

I feel certain that the California State Department of Public Health (fraud division) would provide you with copious data proving you have been poisoning yourselves many hundred years!

Please write soon, and when you do, would you mind telling us why your people are among the healthiest in the world, and why your men and women live vigorous lives well into their 90's, and why you and your beautiful people never get cancer?

Sincerely
Jay Hutchinson.

But reality wasn't funny at all. Because of the controversy and pressure from the establishment against Laetrile, availability of the product was jeopardized. My father, along with other scientists created KEM, S.A. Laboratory in 1972. This institution would supply patients with this extraordinary natural antitumor agent. KEM's Kemdalin is the purest and most effective Laetrile available, according to independent laboratory tests. Today KEM is a trade name for 100% natural pharmaceuticals and supplements; one of the first, and of the few, in the world to stay away completely from synthetic or toxic materials. Dr. Alex Duarte{s book, *The Jaws of Life*, as well as Dr. William Lane{s book, *Sharks Don't Get Cancer*, identify shark cartilage as a powerful supplement with an antiangiogenetic activity which is very beneficial in the destruction of many patient's tumors. ESCUARTROL, Kem's shark cartilage, has been used widely by many.

The following graph shows the results of our Metabolic Therapy in some of the most common malignancies that victimize the population.

AMYGDALIN
Antitumoral Effects

Type of Cancer	No. of Patients	5 year Survival
Prostate	800	87%
Lung	250	30%
Colon	150	30%
Breast (PM)	300	39%

Dr. E. Contreras R.
OASIS Hospital, Tijuana, BC

We must take into consideration that all the patients in these groups had already received treatment with orthodox therapies that had failed them. Their general condition was very poor due to advanced stages of disease. In all of the groups the patients were not expected, statistically, to survive even 6 months. Our results are even more impressive when you take into consideration the results reported in the literature. In the case of patients with inoperable carcinoma of the lung, even when in good condition, the 5 year survival rate is close to zero with orthodox therapies anyway. Patients with prostate cancer can expect a cure rate of around 90% with conventional treatments. This is encouraging but about 66% of them will end up impotent and more than 30% incontinent; with our therapies no side effects. Furthermore, 86% of all patients received important subjective benefits from the treatments. In other words their quality of life improved and they lived much longer than statistically expected. Most oncology researchers don't care about these results, they rather get rid of the tumors -now that is good oncology- unfortunately they also get rid of the patients. I believe that a patient would much rather spend quality time with their families than be tortured and go to the grave sooner; oh yes, but tumor free!

The Solution Lies Within Us All

Undoubtedly the medical industry enjoys a very singular protectionism that allows them to amass fortunes and pile up failures, while cemeteries are reaching the bursting point. It is vital we understand that we must create options to change the devastating trajectory of local and international organizations in charge of our health. Nevertheless, the responsibility is ours alone. I pray that society will demand for doctors to go back to the moral principles worthy of our profession since the authorities, universities and medical associations will not. Only then can we say the words of Hippocrates, with heads held high, and I quote from the original Oath: "So then if I fulfill this oath without fail, may I be granted the enjoyment of life and of my art amid the respect of all men until the end, but if I violate it and perjure myself, may the reverse be my lot ."

- Our health faces serious problems, bombarded by the environment and relegated by the medical industry. Fortunately, there are practical and life saving steps we can take to counteract the aggression from these health adversaries.

Chapter 6

Neither Too Little Nor Too Much

> What is objectionable, what is dangerous, about extremists is not that they are extreme, but that they are intolerant
>
> **Robert Kennedy**

In Chapter Two, we saw how difficult it is to restore the environment and contribute to the reduction of disease. Even if we did begin working individually to do this, it would take decades to make an impact on our health. However, we can easily control the bionomics of our bodies by providing them with adequate, natural nourishment with resources that will help neutralize toxic agents. The internal ecology of our body determines our health.

We eat so that our bodies can have the materials and energy sufficient for existence. In 1750, James Lind was the first to demonstrate scientifically that foods not only have the function of satisfying hunger, but that foods contain essential elements which our bodies can't produce, which determine our physical and mental health. Lind also discovered the relationship between the lack of specific foods and disease. In 1747, he made the first classical study of mariners who suffered from scurvy. For these he prescribed specific foods. Two people who ate oranges and lemons got well in six days. This discovery saved the lives of countless seafaring men who simply began carrying oranges and lemons onboard. In synthesis, this doctor established the impact food has on health. The prophet Hosea proclaimed that people perish due to lack of knowledge. Awareness through information will return our drug oriented culture back to the natural.

The Importance of Nutrients

Insufficient quantities of a nutrient can bring on disease. The lack of a single nutrient can cause death. Lind published his conclusions in 1753 in a work entitled, *A Treatise on Scurvy*. Twenty years had to pass before the findings of Lind made an international impact. At the dawn of chemical science, it took a long time for new discoveries to spread. Remember that in those days there was neither telephone nor telegraph, and no worldwide medical conventions. It was very difficult for information to get from one place to another. The sad thing is that today, in spite of facsimile machines, computers, modems, congresses, and the world wide web, doctors aren't very interested in the wealth of information on nutrition and its impact on our lives.

The era of scientific nutrition began 160 years after Lind's discovery. In 1912, Dr. Casimir Funk discovered thiamin (vitamin B1), and invented the term "vitamin." His discoveries helped cure the disease known as beriberi. Yet, medical science continued to search for miracle drugs instead of applying the advances in nutrition to cardiovascular disease, cancer, diabetes, obesity, arthritis, alcoholism and mental illness. From 1930 to today, extraordinary discoveries continue to be made in the field of essential nutrients. Throughout my medical practice, I have observed that the cancer patients who live the longest are those who indefinitely adhere to a diet based on a high intake of complex carbohydrates (fruits and vegetables), a small intake of animal protein (meats), a minimal intake of animal fat (red meats and milk products) and a vast amount of nutritional supplements. This nutritional plan has a positive impact not only on cancer but on high blood pressure, diabetes, cardiovascular disease, hypercholesterolemia, and just about every other disease.

History has taught us many lessons of this sort but doctors and our industry do not want to accept them, because they cause one to question medical practice as we know it. Advances in technology and the medical sciences have not resolved health problems in the past and will not in the future. We must seriously examine the nutritional, environmental and sociological deficiencies in our communities if we wish to truly resolve health issues. Physicians centuries ago, like Hippocrates and Galen, along with intelligent inventors like Thomas Edison, recommended that proper nutrition would cure better than any medicine. Gladys Block, Ph.D., University of California nutrition researcher, conducted an in-depth analysis of 99 studies to see whether there is actually a connection between diet and cancer. Eighty-nine of the studies disclosed that vegetables and fruit are indeed the first line of defense against many types of cancer.

Thirty-three of the studies show vitamin C and bioflavonoids in berries, cantaloupes, citrus fruits and green leafy vegetables protect us against cancer of the cervix, the esophagus and stomach. Even the skeptical National Cancer Institute recommends eating five servings of fruits and vegetables a day to help prevent cancer.

A Japanese researcher, T. Harayama, conducted a 10 year study of 265,118 subjects who answered questions about their dietary intake. Harayama discovered that people who ate liberal amounts of vegetables containing beta carotene had a lower risk of lung, stomach and prostate cancer.

Finally, the all powerful medical industry with its universities, research laboratories, pharmaceutical factories, sophisticated diagnostic equipment, hospitals and medical societies are a financial success but a disaster to those who put their lives in their hands.

Common diseases like tuberculosis and malaria can make inroads into a body if the general health of the person is poor. Who are the main candidates for disease? People with AIDS, drug addicts, alcoholics, the homeless, and the undernourished. These are the real reasons why, even in countries like the United States, the incidence of infections and other diseases is increasing. For example, a tuberculosis epidemic broke out in a school in Westminster, California, a suburb on the outskirts of Los Angeles. Because of their low income and terrible eating habits, the students there are severely undernourished. Four hundred students contracted tuberculosis form a 16 year old Vietnamese girl! The vast majority responded well to conventional treatments but at least 12 of them had a bacterial strain resistant to antibiotics and continue to deteriorate. One student had to be operated on and lost part of her lung. The better nourished were able to overcome the disease because of a healthy immune system. "The germ is nothing, the terrain is everything."

As I see it, it is necessary to consume very high quantities of nutrients to maintain health. Today many doctors insist (as if they had any idea) that a correctly balanced diet should not demand nutritional supplements. This might have been possible 200 to 300 years ago before the food industry began to heavily manipulate the food supply. Today nutritional supplementing seems both urgent and obligatory. Dr. Yoshihide

Hagiwara, a Japanese Pharmacologists andphysician, developed one of the most powerful whole food concentrates I know, Barleygreen. Barley is a vegetable with outstanding nutritional value that contains chlorophyll, enzymes, minerals, amino acids, vitamins and phytochemicals galore which, on top of providing nutrition, promote detoxification. But, in my opinion, the genius of Dr. Hagiwara's product is what he does to the **soil** where the barley is planted. His premise is that tired and depleted soil (dead soil) produces dead plants. His agriculture specialists prepare the soil with nutrients, not with chemical fertilizers. Of the industrialized countries, the Japanese have the longest life span and that is why I respect their nutritional knowledge and research.

Nutrients Requirements

In the decade of the 1940s, many researchers began to study the variables that determine the individual nutritional needs of a person. Some of these variables were the person's genes, geographic situation, living environment, activity, social context, and state of health. This was a truly titanic task which ended in the futile attempt to make the results practical by recommending daily allowances (RDA) of a given nutrient. In spite of what we have learned about nutrition in the last several decades, people continue to be dazzled by these ridiculous recommendations. It is logical to think that a third rate bureaucrat, whose most intense activity consists of generating an expense report, will require a caloric and nutritional intake infinitely lower than that of a mother with three kids who lives on the fifth floor of an apartment house with no elevator. However, as they eat their corn flakes in the morning, both are totally convinced that they are taking, in one serving, vitamins and minerals sufficient to meet their needs for the day. After all, it says so on the back of the box!

If they were interested, doctors would design a diet based on specific nutritional requirements that take into account the age, gender and health of the individual. I would dare say, however, that this is an impossible task because few doctors are informed about nutrition and they spend so little time with their patients. Instead, nutritionists and dietitians assign pre-established daily requirements which are totally inadequate. This is not too tragic if the patients are healthy but if they are hospitalized, it can be devastating. For example, a patient who has been operated on for a blocked colon has probably not eaten for 48 hours, suffered fever, and lost stored nutrients because of the antibiotics and analgesics taken. In short, the surgical intervention will have caused trauma with a capital T to the body. After the operation the patient usually has to fast. Then, he is given solutions with lots of calories and few nutrients. When the patient can finally eat, he is given gelatin and similar processed foods which increase his need for nutrients. This lack of nourishment provokes severe stress to the system. This is the real reason why some 50,000 deaths occur annually around the United States due to hospital food. Such deaths are directly related to the "diet" prescribed by doctors and dietitians. The ones who do well, do so in spite of the doctor.

The Secret of Balanced Nutrition

In the complex process of keeping our body functioning properly, nutrition supplies the elements necessary to keep 100 trillion cells carrying out their diverse activities. One of the most important activities in the body is the production of replacement cells. This is a vulnerable process because there are many elements that distort genetic information and cause cellular mutations. If the organism has access to adequate resources, it will have the weapons needed to reduce this latent danger. Studies have divided nutrients into two large groups according to the quantities that we need for survival. Those we need in vast quantities are called macronutrients or high volume nutrients. Those we need in small quantities are called micronutrients.

When we speak of nutrients, we immediately think of carbohydrates, proteins and fats. Occasionally we think of a vitamin, yet it is common knowledge that 80% of cellular activity depends directly on these micronutrients. A balanced diet is one that provides sufficient quantities of the macro and micronutrients, although there may be many dietitians and doctors who think that a balanced diet means holding a soft drink in one hand and a cinnamon roll covered with refined sugar in the other. In reality, nearly all foods and vegetables contain both macro and micronutrients, although in different concentrations. For example, the banana is considered to be one of the most perfect foods because it contains all the nutrients needed by the body in the precise amounts needed.

Proteins, carbohydrates and fats are macronutrients. Vitamins, minerals, phytochemicals and enzymes are micronutrients. When we drive our car, what is important to us is that it runs. When we need to pass someone, we want our car to have the power necessary to do so and not falter. We don't stop to think about engine combustion, compression, and temperature. We are only concerned with the car's ability to move. The same thing is true of our body. We want it to run properly. In order to do this it must have energy. We know that we get this energy from food. The macronutrients provide energy called calories. On average, we require 2,000 calories a day. All of these are obtained from carbohydrates, proteins and fats.

MACRONUTRIENTS:
Carbohydrates

Carbohydrates are the main source of energy because they are metabolized easily and quickly. Who has not felt the immediate burst of energy after drinking a glass of orange juice or eating a piece of candy? The waste products they generate are easily eliminated. Carbohydrates are made up of carbon, hydrogen and oxygen. In the liver, they protect liver tissue by helping in the detoxification process. In the heart, they provide the energy that helps the heart contract. In the brain, carbohydrates supply glucose to help regulate the brain's functions.

The vegetable kingdom is the main supplier of carbohydrates. Although they are also found in animals products, the amounts are insignificant. Unfortunately, most people receive around 50% of the needed calories from simple (sugar and flour) carbohydrates. Ideally, we should get 70% of our calories from complex carbohydrates. The most important sources of complex carbohydrates are wheat, rye, corn, potatoes, barley, yucca, grapes, bananas, tomatoes, coconuts, apples, beans, sunflower seeds and mangos.

Proteins

Our body is made up of proteins, the second most abundant substance in the body next to water. These proteins regulate energy production and are instrumental in the building of tissue. Moreover, they are essential in the fight against disease. In a cell, there are thousands of enzymes, all are proteins. Hemoglobin is a protein. Certain hormones like thyroxin, insulin, adrenaline, testosterone, and the estrogens are proteins. All these proteins maintain the smooth functioning of the body.

When we mention the word protein, our imagination turns to beef, pork, poultry, fish, and milk. Yet, these animal proteins are very difficult to process due to the complexity of their molecules and only a small part of them can truly bring benefit to our bodies while the remainder remains as harmful waste. Our bodies break proteins down into amino acids, but the structure of animal proteins requires infinitely more work to break down. For this reason, vegetarians generally live longer than the meat eaters. The easiest proteins to break down are found in grains like wheat, corn, rice, and legumes like beans and lentils. These are followed by the proteins contained in fruits, vegetables and other legumes. Again, the most difficult to break down are those found in animal products.

Amino Acids

Amino acids are the basic building blocks of proteins. They are incredibly versatile elements, uniting to form muscle cells, antibodies, and millions of other things. They have, as the name states, an "amino" side and an "acid" side. This duality is the reason for their biochemical adaptability. Essential amino acids are those that we have to ingest because our bodies cannot produce them. Those that our organism manufactures naturally are called nonessential amino acids; this is one of those semantic scientific blunders because it gives the impression that they are not so important which is totally wrong. The reason we do not have to relay on food to get them is because God felt they were so important that He didn't want to chance their shortage, so He designed the body to produce them on its own. The essential amino acids are isoleucine, leucine, lysine, methionine, phenylalanine, threonine, tryptophan and valine. The nonessential amino acids are alanine, arginine, asparagine, aspartic acid, cysteine, glutamic acid, glutamine, glycine, histidine, proline, serine, and tyrosine. One of the best ways to ease the body's work load is to ingest amino acids instead of proteins.

When wanting to increase one's intake of amino acids, plant sprouts are the best food since they contain large quantities of the essential amino acids. In fact, alfalfa sprouts are the only food containing all the essential amino acids so they should be seen as one of the most complete or perfect foods. Always keep seeds from this super-food; in case you survive the big blast, you could live on alfalfa sprouts and water alone. Granted, after a few months you would start neighing, but most definitively like a **healthy** horse!

Lipids: Fat Has a Bad Rap

Carbohydrates are the main source of quick energy, but fat is one of the most metabolically active of all organic tissues. It constitutes concentrated stored energy. Fats contain more than twice the energy of carbohydrates. When a sufficient number of carbohydrates is lacking, insulin mobilizes the energy concentrated in fatty tissues to supply the needs of the body. Lipids help the body utilize other nutrients like the fat soluble vitamins A, D, E, and K. Fats are not water soluble and their structure is more complex. This is why they are more difficult to digest and assimilate than carbohydrates. Fats also release liposoluble vitamins and essential fatty acids. It can't be denied that fat is essential to life. The problem is that we ingest exorbitant amounts in our present diet. The extra hours spent by the liver digesting animal proteins is nothing compared to the work it must do in the digestion of saturated fats.

Some nutritionists recommend that we not consume more than two tablespoons of fat per day. This includes the oil or butter used to fry foods. This also includes the hidden fats in both processed and natural foods. The people who live the longest consume no more than 10% of their calories from fats.

Saturated Fats

You have undoubtedly heard people speak of saturated fats. They have a uniform configuration. Their acids cluster together compactly and they thus solidify at room temperature. Shortening is the classic example of a saturated fat. Other sources of this type of fat are pork fat, beef tallow, poultry fat, sheep tallow, eggs, milk products, coconut and palm oil. The saturated fats arc considered harmful because it is impossible to metabolize them completely. Saturated fat deposits cause arteriosclerosis, cardiovascular diseases, embolism, and brain hemorrhages. To them we also attribute increases in colon, prostate, and breast cancers, along with metabolic diseases like diabetes.

Unsaturated Fats

Unsaturated fats have a less uniform configuration so they remain in liquid form at room temperature. Foods rich in unsaturated fats include olive oil, corn oil, cottonseed oil, soy oil and peanut oil. When cold pressed, they are a source of essential fatty acids and help improve the quality of the immune system.

Daily Caloric Input

In summary, we ought to get 70% of our calories from carbohydrates, 20% from proteins, and 10% from fats. Yet, to strictly adhere to this measure is difficult because it requires us to limit our choices at each meal. Right now I'm eating a healthy snack that tastes like sawdust. I have to wash it down with mineral water. What I really want is a burrito with beans, refried in lard, and a nice, cold Coke. As St. Paul would say, "Oh miserable man that I am, who shall free me from this body of death?" (Romans 7:24). However, the Bible also says that the "truth" shall make us free, (John 8:32) so let's keep on soaking up authentic information that will enable us to leave bad habits behind and to pursue new ones, even when they are unpleasant.

MICRONUTRIENTS

The micronutrients, as we have already mentioned, are needed by the organism in smaller quantities than the macronutrients. This does not mean, however, that they are not important. On the contrary, they are essential to life.

Vitamins

The word vitamin was invented by Casimir Funk while he was looking for the cause of beriberi. The term vitamin is used to distinguish a nutrient that is neither protein, carbohydrate, fat, nor mineral. Vitamins act mainly as coenzymes. They are not building blocks. They don't produce energy. They are not basic elements, but connectors that affect unions so that organic functions can be attained and maintained within the complex chemical world that is our body. Our health problems would be greatly reduced if we would take vitamins in adequate quantities.

Fruits and vegetables are the most important sources of vitamins. Vitamins improve metabolism, prevent disease and help slow down the aging process. In April 1994, an article appeared in the *New England Journal of Medicine* which dismayed more than a few followers of the principles of good nutrition. The article gave information about a study carried out in Finland with 29,000 smokers who had been taking vitamins E and beta-carotene over periods of five to ten years to discover if they could counteract the risk of lung cancer. At the end of the study, the researchers concluded that the vitamins did not reduce "the total incidence of lung cancer and that the study raised the possibility that these supplements might . . . have dangerous effects as well as beneficial ones." Is this reason to be alarmed?

I agree with the *Newsweek* reporter who stated that, "Although the supplements did not exercise a positive role in the control study reported last week, they can still have a place in the pantry. Strictly interpreted, the latest findings only show that certain vitamins in particular, in certain specific doses, do not reduce the risk of cigarette smoking in Finnish men. Administered in a different way or over a longer period, the same vitamins could produce a different impact." Undoubtedly, the results of these tests are of concern to us but the doses given were ridiculously low. On the other hand, we can't overlook the hundreds of tests that have demonstrated the positive effects of vitamin and nutrient supplements. What we can deduce from the study in Finland is that minimal amounts of vitamins and minerals can't compete with the vast damage caused by the cigarettes. I shall ask Jay Hutchinson to write a letter to the Chinese and Japanese to warn them about the *dangers* of beta carotene and selenium reported; and also ask them why the have such a low incidence of cancer and why the Japanese, that smoke twice as much as the Finnish, have half the incidence of cancer of the lung!

It is certainly true that there is at present a controversy about vitamin supplements. There are studies that demonstrate that "the use of synthetic vitamins (A, B, C, D and E) aggravate the harmful effects of radiation in the offspring of pregnant rats." Big deal! However, other tests prove that nutritional supplements are essential in the prevention of cancer. Research biochemists know it is more than just beta carotene and vitamins C and E in vegetables and fruits that help prevent cancer. Folic acid, one of the B vitamins, is a powerful nutrient, and often deficient in those who need it the most.

Researcher Edward Giovannucci, Harvard Medical School, thinks folic acid may help turn off cancer genes. Giovannucci's team discovered that a high intake of folic acid, from fresh vegetables and fruit and vitamin supplements, lowered the risk of tumor development.

Other research shows folic acid directs the growth of new cells in the body. A shortage or lack of this nutrient may contribute to improper or abnormal cell formation. We now know that a lack of folic acid in early stages of pregnancy increases the chances of birth defects.

Who are we going to believe? The nutritionally challenged minds of the scientists? I personally argue in favor of taking vitamins and other nutritional supplements because we never take in enough of the right foods to obtain the substances needed to prevent disease. The risks that some attribute to the consumption of megadoses of vitamins are unfounded and ludicrous in comparison to the proven risks we run when we don't supplement our diet.

Minerals

The foods the average American eats do not maintain the body's minerals at an adequate level. The human body doesn't have the power to extract minerals directly from the environment nor to manufacture them from other substances. Our only source of mineral provision is food. Minerals allow the body to keep a balance between acidity and alkalinity. Our body requires minerals because it is continuously rebuilding itself. This function is carried out in each one of the cells and the minerals and vitamins act as catalyzing agents in the process. When these catalysts are lacking, the biochemical reactions are carried out in an incomplete way, forming toxic products that slow down the regenerative process.

> And the Lord God formed man from the dust of the ground, and breathed into his nostrils the breath of life; and man became a living soul.
>
> **Genesis 2:7**

We were created from the dust, thus all the materials that form us are in the soil or earth. Of the elements most important for our organs to function and survive, minerals are at the top of the list and we obtain them, directly or indirectly, from the soil. No plant or animal survives without them.

The planets and stars are made of them and we humans desperately need them in our earthly bodies.

Among the vegetables that best provide minerals are broccoli, spinach, water cress, coriander, lettuce, parsley, sweet peppers, tomatoes, chili peppers, prickly pears, and mushrooms.

USA government surveys confirm that the average American diet provides only 40% of the recommended daily amount of magnesium. In a two-year Food and Drug Administration study to analyze 234 foods, they found the average American diet to have less than 80% of the recommended daily allowance (RDA) of one or more of these minerals: calcium, magnesium, iron, zinc, copper and manganese. What's worse is that RDAs are sadly insufficient for maintaining health.

A large study conducted by the USA Department of Agriculture found that only 25% of 37,785 individuals had magnesium intakes at or greater than the RDA, which is notoriously low. A 1995 review of 15 studies found that a typical diet contains only a fraction of RDA.

Maurene Kennedy Salaman, author of *Foods That Heal*, *Nu-*

trition: The Cancer Answer II and the soon-to-be-released book *Encyclopedia of Natural Healing,* among other books, is an authority on the subject of minerals. She recommends *Maximum Living's MINERAL RICH,* a mineral solution supplemental formula, because, "Science has shown that minerals dissolved in water are more bio-available than those present in food," she points out. I agree with her assessment that "Taking minerals in solution will overcome any of the limitations you might have that inhibit your ability to absorb them. A patent-pending process, called the *Solucell method,* adds to the benefit as it causes the minerals to be quickly and completely absorbed into the bloodstream, restoring gaps that could lead to illness and disease."

Enzymes

Enzymes are proteins produced by our genes. They are the most important and powerful of the molecules because they carry out all the chemical changes that take place within the cells. They facilitate the breaking down and synthesis of food in the digestive tract.

The additional functions of enzymes are extremely broad. For example, in the mouth, enzymes break down starches into complex carbohydrates. In the stomach, they convert proteins into amino acids and complex carbohydrates into simple carbohydrates.

In the small intestine, enzymes convert fats into fatty acids. When our body suffers an injury, they help stop hemorrhage and they promote the creation of new cells. At present, some 3000 enzymes are known and it is crucial that we ingest an adequate supply of them.

Fiber

Fibers are substances our organism can't digest or metabolize. They are most commonly found in the vegetable kingdom. Fibrous substances are lodged in the external layers that protect the seeds and fruits. Perhaps the best known fiber is bran which encases cereal grains. Fiber presents a rough texture that serves to defend the grain from external destructive agents. It is precisely this protective aspect of fiber that allows it to pass through our body unaltered. Fiber helps eliminate waste that accumulate in the digestive tract. It helps solidify diarrhea and loosen constipation. It drags along with it potentially harmful substances and helps detoxify the organism. It helps maintain the volume and softness of intestinal content, as well as reduce the internal pressure related to diverticular diseases. The lack of raw fiber in the diet produces constipation, colonic irritation, appendicitis, hemorrhoids, varicose veins, colon and many other cancers, gallstones, obesity, diabetes, and high blood cholesterol. Fiber is a food essential to the preservation of good health not because of its nutritional contribution, but because of its physiological properties. It keeps the digestive system in good order.

Antioxidants

We have already noted in Chapter One the devastating effects of oxidation caused by free radicals. Nutrition writer Patrick Quillin, Ph.D., calls these vicious molecules, "Great white sharks in the biochemical sea of life." These cell saboteurs have long been suspected of triggering various cancers and other diseases.

To a great degree, the state of our health will depend on the capacity we have to neutralize free radicals and stop their destructive action. Cells have the ability to produce neutralizers called antioxidants. Our body produces its own antioxidants but the consumption of certain foods can provide additional antioxidants, giving additional protection against the destructive impact of such free radicals. Among other nutrients, the most outstanding antioxidants are the vitamins C, E and beta-carotene. Selenium is an antioxidant mineral essential to any program of cancer preventive care. Make sure it is part of your arsenal, and is combined with all the other minerals. Other potent free-radical fighting supplements are coenzyme Q10, SOD (superoxide dismutase), and vitamin B17, otherwise known as Laetrile and Amygdalin.

In theory, if we are able to neutralize free radicals, we can diminish the incidence of disease and slow the aging process. Dr. John P. Richey, Jr. of the School of Medicine of Louisville University uses antioxidants to prolong the average life span of rats up to 64%. Researchers reported that "a recent analysis of 170 studies carried out in 17 different countries reveal that people who consume the most fruits and vegetables present cancer rates some 50% lower than those who consume these elements in lower quantities." The elements in the fruits and vegetables responsible for this are the antioxidants and phytochemicals. In double blind studies by Dr. Harmon, originator of the theory of aging by free radicals, it was discovered that the antioxidants have an anti-tumoral effect. There are many foods that are rich in antioxidants and phytochemicals. Phytochemicals are neither vitamins nor minerals, yet they are equally potent and vital to the healthy functioning of our bodies. They are isolated from plants and are known technically as anthocyanosides, limonoids, glucarates, phenolic acids, flavonoids, coumarins, polyacetylenes and carotenoids.

Phytochemicals throw a biochemical wrench into one or more of the mechanisms leading to tumor development. "At almost every one of the steps along the pathway leading to cancer," says epidemiologist John Potter of the University of Minnesota, "there are one or more compounds in vegetables or fruits that slow or reverse the process". The following is a list of these foods and their benefits.

- Broccoli, cauliflower, Brussels sprouts, turnips, kale, turnip greens and bok choy are the most highly-re garded anti-cancer foods. Researches have isolated a chemical in them called **sulforaphane** as responsible for their cancer preventive properties.

- Cabbage and turnips contain another anti-cancer ingre dient, acronymed **PEITC**. Gary Stoner of Ohio State, reports that PEITC inhibits lung cancer in mice and rats.

- **Ellagic acid**, found in strawberries, grapes and raspberries, also neutralizes carcinogens before they can invade DNA.

- Garlic and onions contain **allylic sulfides** which protect against cancer of the stomach. They have multiple phytochemicals that diminish "bad" cholesterol and elevate the "good," reducing the risk of cardiovascular diseases. I will talk more about garlic ahead.

- Soybeans contain **genistein**. This phytochemical has an anti-aggregate that won't allow small tumors to attach themselves to capillaries. In this way, the tumors can't get nutrients and, consequently, they can't metastasize. They also contain phytohormones with the "good" estrogenic action without the undesirable effects of the synthetic estrogens.

- Chili peppers contain the phytochemical **capsaicin**, which does not allow the carcinogens in cigarette smoke to penetrate the DNA. Thus, the carcinogens can't trigger the mutations that produce lung and other cancers.

- Citrus fruits and blackberries contain **flavonoids** and prevent carcinogenic hormones from being introduced into the cells. Of course, almost all fruits and vegetables contain these anticancer phytochemicals.

- Tomatoes, strawberries, pineapple and dried chili contain the phytochemicals **p-coumaric acid** and **chlorogenic acid** that block the marriage of molecules that form carcinogens.

- Red and yellow - not white - onions contain an incredible amount of **quercetin** - 10% or more of their dry weight. Various lab studies reveal that quercetin unleashes a one-two punch against cancer, it blocks cell changes that invite cancer and, if a tumor has already started, it stops the spread of malignant cells.

- Cassava, bitter almonds, apricot pits, lentils, millet, beans and sweet potatoes all contain a tremendously beneficial phytochemical, **Amygdalin**, also called vitamin B17, which is the crown jewel in the extrinsic nutritional defense mechanism against cancer.

Amounts of Fruits and Vegetables for Cancer Prevention

Five or more servings of fruits and vegetables daily will help to prevent cancer. A serving equals one-half cup of fruit or vegetables, a cup of raw leafy vegetables, a medium-sized piece of raw fruit, or 170 grams of fruit or vegetable juice. It is best to eat the fruit and vegetables raw. Cooking destroys nutrients, except phytochemicals, which are not affected in the preparation of food.

Scientists recently found that people in northern Italy who ate seven or more servings of raw tomatoes (containing the phytochemical lycopene) every week had 60% less chance of developing colon, rectal and stomach cancer than those who ate two servings or less.

Cornell University researchers reported that two tomatoes contain an estimated 10,000 phytochemicals including: p-coumaric acid and chlorogenic acid, which stop the formation of cancer-causing substances. Tomato acids remove the nitrosamines before they can do any damage. Cornell's Joseph Hotchkiss gave volunteers tomato juice and found less nitrosamines in their bodies.

Herbert Pierson, PH.D., former project director with the National Cancer Institute, says that bioflavonoids enhance the body's detoxification system, protect cell membranes, and help regulate enzymes that go unchecked when a cell becomes malignant. Almost every fruit and vegetable, from berries to yams to citrus and cucumbers, contain bioflavonoids. In a cellular version of musical chairs, bioflavonoids race to sites on the cell where cancer-causing hormones, including estrogen, attach themselves. When the music stops, the bioflavonoids keep the hormones from sitting down on the cell's surface. This is especially important regarding the role of estrogen in breast cancer.

Dr. Terence Leighton, a biochemistry professor at the University of California, Berkeley, is a world authority on phytochemicals and believes that, "Quercetin is one of the strongest anti-cancer agents known."

Anti-cancer enzymes, found only in whole fruits, vegetables and grains, are what make the difference between people who get cancer and those who don't. You need enough free-floating enzymes in your system to conquer cancer every day!

Enzymes are needed for the body to use many nutrients, especially proteins. More than two thousand varieties play vital roles in every human physical function. Historically, enzyme therapy has been used in cancer treatment successfully for decades.

Dr. Paul Talalay, of Johns Hopkins Medical Institute, added the phytochemical sulforaphane to human cells growing in a lab dish and reported that it boosted the growth of anti-cancer enzymes. In April 1994 issue of *Proceedings of the National Academy of Sciences,* his team reported conclusively that the compound protects living animals against cancer.

We should be eager to eat fruits and vegetables, since we automatically benefit from the protective qualities of their phytochemicals, but supplementation with products like Preven-Ca, Barleygreen and other quality products is advisable.

Alkaline Water

We can assist phytochemicals by drinking alkaline substances which provide negative ions. In Chapter One, we spoke about the dangers of failing to maintain a proper pH. I don't believe that there is any bodily process more sophisticated than the maintenance of an adequate level of pH in the blood. pH measures the acidity and alkalinity of our body and all of its fluids. The level of pH in the blood must be meticulously controlled. Blood pH should be at 7.4, and a pH lower than 7.1 or higher than 7.9 can cause death.

The pH scale runs from 0 to 15, with 0 meaning the most acidic, and 15 the most alkaline. The proper pH level is neutral - neither acid nor alkaline - but standing at the center of the scale at 7.4 to 7.5. Our body keeps our blood's pH neutralized in an extremely effective way. Blood pH is constantly affected by the environment, especially by toxins introduced to the body when we eat or drink. Think of cola drinks, which are very acidic. To neutralize the acid in a glass of soda, we would need to mix it with 32 glasses of water. Thirty-two glasses of water? What happens to our bodies? Why doesn't a soda damage us immediately unless we drink 32 glasses of water to neutralize it? In the face of such an emergency situation, the body makes use of a process called ionization. When blood is acidified, it has an overabundance of hydrogen ions (H). The blood then produces hydroxyl (OH) which unites with these ions, producing water (H_2O). Water has a neutral pH of 7.4. In order for the process of ionization to work efficiently, enormous quantities of oxygen are consumed with obvious negative impact on our health. Another way to maintain proper pH is to eat large quantities of alkaline substances to counteract all the acids we consume. Alkaline substances are formed from foods that produce negative ions like spinach, soy, carrots, mushrooms, potatoes, radishes, cucumbers, onions, bananas, and fruits. Yet another method is to drink mineral water or alkali water, which can be prepared in water ionizers. Barleygreen is the highest alkaline food tested.

Factors That Influence Nutrition

How wonderful if the solution to all our health problems was as easy as following all the previously mentioned recommendations. Unfortunately, many people who follow these guidelines still experience disease. In order to preserve good health, it is necessary to maintain the body's natural balance called homeostasis. This balance is arrived at by absorbing from food all the energy necessary for survival and eliminating all toxic waste in order to prevent disease. Yet, there are a number of factors that effect the body's ability to maintain this homeostasis.

Hormones

Molecular biologists are working to discover the cause of aging at the genetic level. In 1990, Dr. Daniel Rudman, an endocrinologist, tried to hold back the effects of aging in men between 60 and 70 years old. Rudman utilized growth hormones in his experiments. This hormone helps form scar tissue, reinforces the immune system, strengthens bones, builds muscle, repairs organs, and helps the body break down fat. Rudman gathered a group of 21 men together. To half of them he gave a synthetic version of growth hormone three times a week. To the other half he gave nothing. He performed monthly examinations to note the manifestations of aging in all the men. The men treated with hormones recuperated 10% of their muscle, the skin increased its thickness by 9% and they lost 14% of their body fat. The livers and spleens of these men recovered mass. Some of the men felt mild pain in their hands due to an increase of muscle mass and the pressure it created on the joints. But in general, almost all reported noticeable improvements, compared to the group that received no hormones. When the experiment was over, and the men stopped taking the growth hormones, they lost the youthful qualities they had gained.

Rudman's experiment demonstrated that more than one factor is involved in aging. There are a whole host of hormones that affect the aging process. At 45 years of age, men produce lower quantities of testosterone and the general state of their health often deteriorates. If these men receive testosterone injections their sexual impulse increases, their muscles are strengthened, and they fight anemia more effectively. Another hormone that helps slow down the aging process is the adrenal hormone, dehydroepiandrostrone (DHEA). The body converts it into other hormones related to the sexual impulse, immune system and memory. It prevents obesity, diabetes and arteriosclerosis. In our youth, our bodies produced this hormone in great abundance. At age 30, this production begins to diminish. This is one of the reasons why people tend to gain weight more easily as they advance in age. A deficiency of DHEA can cause breast cancer and heart attacks. Melatonin is another "mother hormone," our body will convert into any hormone that it needs at that time.

Hormone replacement therapy (HRT) is going through a positive change. More and more physicians diminishing dosages of estrogen they prescribe for menopause. The use of natural progesterone and phyto-estrogens that prevent female cancers are gaining popularity. Good sources of natural hormones can be found in Mexican wild yam creams and concentrates of soy which are now readily available to the public. These are only a few examples of the powerful impact hormones have on the aging process.

Quality Produces Quality

It is possible to obtain these hormones and slow aging but to date, it has been difficult. What is more within our ability to control is the food we eat. The quality, density and variety of the food we eat is important but their effectiveness depends on the nutrients getting to the place where they are needed. We have already remarked on how foods degenerate due to environmental, industrial and processing factors. There are things that keep nutrients from getting to where they are desperately needed. We don't chew our food enough, or give it sufficient time to mix with saliva. Saliva contains multiple enzymes absolutely essential to good digestion. The next step involves the absorption of nutrients through the mucous-covered intestinal lining and the subsequent transfer to the bloodstream and the liver. This organ has the incredible task of feeding our cells. Each type of cell has its own distinct needs. So, the liver functions like a cook, attending to some 100 trillion finicky customers. This process is crucial if we are to maintain good health. Yet, there are hundreds of obstacles that keep nutrients from strengthening the body. If we don't chew well, if the stomach is irritated by gastritis, if there are absorption problems in the intestine, if the chemical processes of digestion are deficient, if the intestinal flora has been destroyed by some antibiotic, if the liver is in no condition to metabolize food, if the arteries are coated on the inside with cholesterol and restrict the passage of nutrients to the cells, if the cellular membrane isn't prepared to utilize the nutrients, and if there are medicines that intercept the nutrients, this process is obstructed. The body must overcome these complicated obstacles to maintain good health. It is up to us to facilitate this troublesome task.

Obesity

In Mexico, around 70% of the population is obese. In the United States, about 71% are obese. These figures sound impossible because we don't observe a lot of very fat people in public. We believe that an obese person is someone who weighs more than 200 pounds. However, if a person's body weight exceeds their ideal weight by 20%, they are obese. Why is it that the magical 20% of excess weight is considered to be obesity? Because statistically, people with this level of excess weight have a disease related mortality rate between 20% and 40% higher than those who don't have this extra weight. Therefore, one of the most urgent problems that modern society must solve is that of obesity.

Obesity can also be viewed as an excess of toxins in the organism. The human body was designed to maintain a balance between the building of tissues and the tearing down of them. When one of these processes takes place in excess, it causes metabolic imbalance. The body is constantly replacing old cells with new. Between 300 billion and 800 billion old cells are replaced by others every day. Dead cells should be eliminated through the intestines, bladder, lungs, or skin. In the obese, this process is less efficacious and the body finds itself affected by the retention of toxins. Toxins also form because the organism was designed to digest natural foods. When processed foods are eaten they give more work to the digestive apparatus, causing incomplete digestion and toxic build-up.

Besides this, toxins are acidic in nature. When acids accumulate in the body, the system retains water to neutralize them. This causes weight increase and swelling. If more toxins are generated than the body can eliminate, the body stores them primarily in adipose fat and in the lumen of our arteries as cholesterol. This is one of the main causes of arteriosclerosis, which is in turn one of the primary producers of heart attacks, embolisms, and other vascular diseases which are the main cause of death in developed countries.

People perceive eating as a pleasurable activity only, forgetting that the main goal of eating is the nourishment of the body. Consider that the brain control appetite by the concentration of nutrients in the blood and cells and not caloric "deficiency." If we satisfy hunger with a big-high-calorie-hamburger, we will be full but in a short time hungers strikes again -for lack of nutrients -so we eat a pizza! When we consume nutritious food, hunger attacks are going to spread apart. This means, among other things, maintaining an ideal weight.

We consume on average 5000 calories a day; about 2500 more than required by the average person. We foolishly believe that doing 10 more minutes of exercise will burn the extra calories of the second serving we ate. Exercise burns calories, yes, but not as many as we would like; bicycling for an hour burns less than 130 calories, advanced single tennis players consume 650 calories in one hour. That's not very comforting when a single slice of pecan pie has more than 500 calories.

Most westerners (70%) have a weight problem. I breathe and gain a pound! Of course there are some people that don't have to worry about it. I have a friend that eats as if that meal was going to be his last one and never gains any weight. When you are making all efforts to maintain your weight (eating like a rabbit, watching every calorie, skinning your minute piece of organically grown chicken, exercising, etc.) facing nevertheless, a loosing battle to stay in that already-tight-clothing size, he's the typical guy you want to strangle! Yes, most of us suffer from the battle of the bulge.

But Chinese, that eat rural and primitive diets, consume more calories than us and rarely will you see an obese person in China (unless he is an American tourist). Why? It is because they have not obstructed their "thermogenetic" mechanism. The invasion of our environment and food with hormones, and hormone-like substances, has deteriorated an intrinsic mechanism by which our body burns excess calories: thermogenesis.

Thermogenesis means literally - generation of heat. In metabolic terms, it's the mechanism by which calories are converted into heat rather than accumulated in white fat. This important regulatory function is performed at the level of the mitochondria of the brown adipose tissue (BAT).

Thermogenesis can be restored naturally by consumption of nutrients and herbs that stimulate adrenergic transmitters that activate the "uncoupling protein" (only present in BAT) that derails the normal conversion of calories into ATP (energy) to heat. Ephedra and Salix are plants that specifically stimulate BAT. Many criticize their use because they could be toxic, but these plants are not toxic. When the active ingredients are extracted and used as single agents, they can cause symptoms like anxiety, tachicardia (fast heart rate), and hypertension; but when taken in harmony with the rest of the phytochemicals of the plants, the adverse effects are completely neutralized.

At KEM labs, we developed a product with 100% natural plants that regenerate thermogenesis called KEM-A KLIOS, which means "pound burner." In a double blind study, 100 obese subjects were given the product, they were not required to make any changes in their life style. After 6 months, 70% of the ones who took the thermogenetic herbal product, KEM-A-KILOS, lost between 30% and 90% of their excess weight, but more importantly almost all reported going to a smaller dress size. None of the patients reported any adverse effects except that they had more energy and had to spend money on new, smaller clothes. In the placebo group, only 12% lost weight

Reducing body weight equals increased energy, self-esteem, and reduced risk of disease. The closer you are to your ideal weight, the less chances you have of acquiring diseases like cancer, cardiovascular, diabetes and many other. Poor and excessive eating habits are obviously the cause of weight gain but another problem is that we are too sedentary. Exercise plays an important role in the health of the body, too. There is nothing like exercise to make our body function better.

Exercise

Chauncey Depew, an American politician, said that he got his exercise "acting as a pallbearer to his friends who exercise." Most of us don't even begin to exercise because we think we need to do a lot of it to make a difference. A friend of mine is convinced that the secret to her abundant health is that whenever the impulse to exercise comes over her, she lies down until it passes away!

The fact is that little exercise is needed to get more out of our bodies. One of the easiest and most accessible exercises is walking. To keep yourself in good physical condition, you should, on average, walk briskly from 25 to 60 minutes 3 times a week; that's not asking much at all! All exercise reduces the chemical stress by the neutralization of acids. Beyond that, exercise promotes many other mechanisms that generate health and long life. The following is a short list of the benefits provided by exercise.

- The Central Nervous System: Exercise improves mental agility and memory, rehabilitates disturbances of the nervous system, improves sexual vigor.

- The Skeletal and Muscular System and The Skin: Exercise keeps skin firm and more pliable, improves posture, reduces dysfunction of the joints, improves flexibility, strengthens the bones, fortifies the musculature, improves equilibrium, is important in the rehabilitation of auto-immune diseases (for example, rheumatoid arthritis and muscular dystrophy), and isessential to post-traumatic rehabilitation (wounds and accidents).

- The Metabolic, Digestive and Excretory Systems: Exercise increases basal metabolism, helps control the metabolism of sugars, reduces body fat, increases muscular volume, prevents constipation and its concomitant disorders.

- The Cardiovascular and Respiratory Systems: Exercise improves the efficiency of the heart and lungs, increases circulation, reduces cholesterol, reduces high blood pressure, expands lung capacity and is basic to rehabilitation programs after heart attacks and cerebral embolisms.

- The Psychological and Immune Systems: Exercise strengthens the immune system, reduces depression, helps in the psychological battle against disease, lifts the spirits, helps control addictions to cigarettes, alcohol and caffeine and improves self-esteem.

Undernourishment

The inhabitants of developed countries think that undernourishment is rare because we associate the word with places with famines like Biafra, Bangladesh, and Somalia. There are many types of malnutrition, but for now I will talk about the lack of nutrients. Lack of nutrients is attributed to low intake of food or the intake of inadequate foods (which some call malnutrition). Whatever the cause of the lack of nourishment in the organism may be, doctors tend to forget that sickness is often closely related to malnutrition. Sadly enough, there are thousands of people who die every day because they don't have food. Equally unfortunate is the fact that thousands die of malnutrition. They have too much to eat of those expensive nutritionally empty foods. For example, in the United States, 70% of all deaths are related to excessive consumption of fat, sugar and salt. The majority of elderly people over 60 suffer from deficiency of vitamins A, B12, C, calcium and iron. The population in general suffers from deficiency in zinc, folic acid, vitamin C, vitamin B6, copper, calcium and iron. On the other hand, the consumption of salt is universally excessive.

In Mexico, on June 19, 1994, the newspaper *La Jornada* published the following note, "Twenty-four million Mexicans are below the minimum levels of nutrition," we are assured by Faviano Dominguez, Coordinator of the Program for the Promotion of Health of the Mexican Social Security Institute. He further explains that these unbalanced eating habits provoke high infant mortality as well as causing irreparable damage in the physical and mental development of children. Mexico has a total population of 95 million. Undernourishment is, albeit indirectly if you wish, a factor in the stagnation of the development of a country. Let's take into account that a prolonged deficiency of nutrients brings as a consequence a slowing of growth, productivity, libido, vigor, energy, and appetite. How can a country produce or be creative if its inhabitants don't have the vitality for it? What quality of life can these people have? It's like an architect who is assigned a project and has to adapt to a budget. If he is given sufficient elements to build a quality building, it is possible for him to build it. If he can only count on bad materials, his building will be of inferior quality. So it is with our organism which almost imperceptibly, marvelously adapts itself to the changing patterns of its DNA to produce cells in harmony with the nutritive budget made available. But different from architectural plans, our organism passes genetic information on to succeeding generations and so perpetuates a race with deficiencies. Poor nutrition lowers fertility and affects pregnancy, producing high mortality and damaging physical development. A country of undernourished and obese people is a country without energy. If adequate nutrition means anything, it means health energy.

Food Preparation

The discovery of fire revolutionized life in many ways but I think that its greatest impact was on food. It seems very interesting to me that tribes in all parts of the world have developed incredibly similar ways of preparing foods involving the use of fire. Bread, for example, is a universal food that is baked. In addition, a fair number of foods can't be made without preparation in the kitchen. Some examples are grains and cereals. It is necessary to clean and disinfect others of dirt and pesticides.

A few decades ago people bought daily what was needed for daily consumption. The modern homemaker goes to the market two or three times a month. The storing of food is at present an integral part of our existence but let's remember that organic foods keep their nutrients for only a few days after harvesting. Foods stay fresh in the refrigerator for about eight days. It is good, therefore, to buy vegetables and fruits to be consumed as soon as possible. In these difficult times, we neither want nor should waste anything so prepare only what is needed but if something is left over, keep it covered so as not to lose any more nutrients. We should not allow foods to spoil, lest we turn the refrigerator into a bacteria culture chamber.

Like all things that evolve and progress, the process of attaining these goals have their price. Now flavor reigns over nutrients. Utensils have evolved too. Of the clay and wooden ones, nothing remains; they have been replaced by more durable instruments. Nevertheless, many utensils are dangerous to health. Part of the Mexican tradition is cooking in clay pots but it has been discovered that the clay contains lead. Aluminum utensils are also harmful because they form aluminum salts that coat the inside walls of the digestive system and impede the formation of normal digestive secretions. Aluminum can cause ulcers and cancer. Beyond that, aluminum is introduced into the bloodstream and added to fatty and brain tissues increasing the risk of Alzheimer's disease.

Another material that definitely affects our health is teflon. The pans safe for cooking are made of glass, enameled cast iron and stainless steel. Cook your food in utensils in good condition, not ones that are chipped or rusted because these contaminate food and there is already too much of that in the environment.

I sincerely hope this information helps you to acknowledge that you have to change your unhealthy habits. But if not, at least it should stop you from enjoying them!

Recommendations To Help Your Body Get More From Nutrients

It is clearly our responsibility to keep our body in the best possible condition. Sadly, no one talks to us about the destructive vices of eating non-natural contaminated foods which we should avoid. If you don't believe this, this book will make no sense. Knowledge alone is worthless, I hope that what you have learned can be put to practice; wisdom that surely we can achieve. Solomon said that "the beginning of wisdom is the fear of the Lord." You may ask what does that have to do with what I should eat? Or how often should I move my bowels? The fear of the Lord has nothing to do with being afraid of Him, it has everything to do with respecting Him as the creator. Creation requires law to maintain order. We are, like it or not, still subject to the rules of the game. In other words, the laws of nature will fall on us with all their force.

> But if ye will not hearken unto me, and will not do all these commandments; (Lev 26:14) ...I also will do this unto you; I will even appoint over you terror, consumption, and the burning ague, that shall consume the eyes, and cause sorrow of the heart: and ye shall sow your seed in vain...(Lev 26:16);... I will send the pestilence among you...(Lev 26:25).

If we respect Him, all will go well. If not, we will suffer the consequences. God can override His rules, that's why there are exceptions, but normally the rules stick.

The Good Old Fashion Way

Thanks to public awareness in the last decade, U.S. citizens have finally begun modifying their eating habits. They have replaced the classic breakfast of eggs, bacon and coffee with fruit, cereal and juice. But more importantly, food production is experiencing a refreshing change.

I know of a cattleman in Colorado who decided to retire from business and was left with a few head of cattle he couldn't sell. He didn't want to kill them so he let them loose in a field to eat pure pasture. A few months later, he was surprised when someone offered him a very attractive price for his stock. He couldn't believe that they were interested in buying tough meat that had been untreated with hormones. Now this cattleman is the largest producer of organic cattle in the United States. He lets his stock graze over unsprayed pastures and he doesn't use any growth hormones or antibiotics. Today, it is increasingly easier to find organic beef and chicken. In addition, agricultural companies which produce organic fruits and vegetables are on the rise. For example, Walnut Acres in Philadelphia provides some 700 tons of organically grown produce to the marketplace each year. Their production has increased in each of the last five years and annual sales are approaching 8 million dollars. To date, there are 100 supermarkets in the United States that offer their products. The sale of natural products has changed from a health nut binge to a leading movement in the industry, according to

Paul Keene, founder of Walnut Acres. The availability of organically grown food is increasing. As more of us begin to consume natural products, we will enjoy healthier lives and save our planet at the same time.

Here are some recommendations, simple and easy to follow, that can affect the quality of our life in profoundly beneficial ways.

- Take Enough Time To Eat: The fast pace of our lives often causes us to skip a meal here and there. The concept of priority is definitely the most vague in human life and it is likely to be so in reference to our eating habits. Eating takes time. So, make time for it. The **right kind of food** in the right sized serving must be eaten in a reasonable amount of time.

- Make Food A Pleasant Social Event: All human beings relate better to each other when they partake of food. During mealtime our body heals itself and supplies energy for itself. If nutrients hit the bloodstream when the body is loaded with adrenaline, a hormone that abounds when we are frightened or angry, the utilization of nutrients is impeded. For this reason, I recommend that you relax before you eat. If you are under stress, take a few minutes to calm down and take some deep breaths before the meal.

- Chew Food Very Well: Another step very much within our reach is to chew very thoroughly before swallowing food. This will facilitate digestion for two reasons. One, the foods are finely ground. Practice chewing each bite 30 times. Not only will you feel better, you will eat less and feel more satisfied. Also, this will assure a better moistening of the food with saliva which causes the action of the gastric juices to be more effective. Some enzymes are activated or release when food is broken or crunched as well.

- Choose Not To Ingest Liquid During Meals: Normally, we use drinks to help us swallow our food. However, this keeps the digestive mechanism from segregating gastric juices, especially if the drinks are extremely cold or hot. If food is well chewed, we don't need drinks. A small glass of water before or after a meal is sufficient. We must drink at least eight large glasses of water during the day but not at mealtime. The water should be consumed between meals and upon rising and before retiring.

- Don't Eat Too Much: I again emphasize the matter of not eating excess quantities of animal products, refined flours and fats. Stay away from alcoholic beverages which are notorious for depleting nutrients. Volunteers who had two alcoholic drinks daily turned out to have an 85% higher risk of developing tumors than non-drinkers. This recommendation is also applied to vegetables and fruits. Excess of any sort of food overload alters the functioning of the digestive system.

The Hunza and natives of other cultures used to say that one should not eat more than what will sit in two cupped hands.

- Give Yourself Time For Excretion: Not that you need a newspaper, a magazine and the Bible because of constipation. If you eat correctly, defecation should be a pleasure. Defecation is a function vital to health. Constipation is often caused because we don't give ourselves enough time for excretion, in other words, we postpone the urge for a more "convenient" time. In our present society, it is seen as poor taste and embarrassing to excuse ourselves to go to the toilet. For this reason, it has been taught that it is best to have a fixed time for excretion, either in the morning or in the evening, so as not to be chagrined. But really, just as we drink water when we are thirsty and eat when are hungry, we should defecate when we feel the need. It is a good idea to eat fiber and try to excrete waste three times a day.

- Nutrient supplementation cannot be stressed enough; thank God more and more companies are coming out with quality products. One that I recommend, as I have already mentioned is Barleygreen because it not only provides powerful nutritional value, it has wonderful, natural cleansing agents that help each and every cell function better. Dr. Mary Ruth Swope, a major proponent of AIM International's Barleygreen, shares in her book, *Green Leaves Of Barley*, "The juice from green barley leaves is definitely one of the best general detoxifiers. It's full of flavonoids which detoxify

the cellular tissue as well as polypeptides which can neutralize nicotine and heavy metals, like mercury, into
soluble salts. Everything about it helps to strengthen the
mechanisms that purge the bloodstream and excrete the
toxins."

Better quality and longer life await the ones that make the
sacrifices recommended in this book, but I remind my "heath
nut" friends that always carry their tupper-ware full of sprouts
and organically grown veggies, policing everything everybody
else eats, that the clothes they are wearing have at least 7000
toxic chemicals, not even in our graves are we free of toxins!

Because of the devastating effect our environment has on our
bodies and the increasing contact we have with carcinogens,
we have developed a product that will counter toxins' damage
with a multitude of powerful phytochemicals found in a number of natural, wild (organic) plants and shark cartilage. KEM
laboratories produces this supplement called Preven-CA, The
combination of herbs consists of alfalfa, milk thistle, boldus,
grape seeds, carrot, and garlic.

Another supplement I recommend is Vita-Sprout, from Maximum Living, a product that uses the sprouts and vegetables
highest in phytochemicals, antioxidants, enzymes, vitamins
and minerals which have been freeze-dried during their most
nutritionally active phase to create a formula high in cancer
preventive nutrients.

If all the recommendations I have given you seem impossible or unrealistic, I'll give you one you cannot refuse: Consume garlic. Now-a-days you don't have to isolate yourself or be afraid to lose your love life. There are many products with odorless garlic.

Garlic, the monarch of the vegetable kingdom, is a leader that has many qualities and powers, because of them it has been used for medicinal purposes since the ancient Egyptians. But the early Greeks, Chinese, Japanese and Mayans also favored this incredible root. Dioscorides, chief physician for the Roman army in the year 200 said "garlic doth cleared the arteries." The beneficial effects that garlic has for the human race are wide and dependable.

Although the virtues of garlic, a side from the culinary, have been accepted for years, only recently scientists have "discovered" some of its royal attributes. Garlic is known to have therapeutical value in a wide variety of diseases. From an antibiotic (as potent as penicillin or tetracycline), anti micotic (fungus), anti viral, to cancer killing powers.

One quality researched is the ability to elevate the capacity of our immune system. The University of Loma Linda, and the John Wayne Cancer Institute, both in California, have gathered data that unequivocally demonstrates the immense immune capabilities of Aged Garlic Extract. Dr. Abdullah from the Akbar Clinic and Research Foundation in Panama City, Florida (go figure), reported at the 5th AIDS International

Conference in Quebec, Canada (1989), that garlic increased the natural killer cell activity in patients with AIDS.

The State University of New York reported that garlic improved the condition of arteriosclerotic arteries through inhibition of the abnormal growth and multiplication of arterial lining cells. Dr. Manfred Steiner, a Hematologist at Memorial Hospital, Brown University in Rhode Island, published that garlic has compounds with potent inhibitors of platelet adhesion. So cardiovascular disease patients, on top of increasing their immune systems, when they take garlic they lower their cholesterol, greatly reduce their incidence of dying from a heart attack, and don't need to take coumadin, a blood thinning drug that, by the way, is also used as rat poison!

The National Cancer Institute, Cornell University Medical College and Memorial Sloan Kettering have reported that garlic inhibits the growth of human breast cancer; other reports establish inhibiting effects against bladder, colon, skin and lung cancer. It has also been demonstrated that it has a powerful detoxification action and that it is a relieving adjutant to chemotherapy, helping patients diminish its side effects.

The scientific research of garlic has been done, in most part (80%), by Wakunaga Pharmaceuticals, a Japanese company. Even though garlic cannot be patented, they have sponsored terribly expensive research in institutes around the world.

They have certainly used the excellent results to promote their Aged Garlic Extract, Kyolic, but at the same time it helps their competitors increase their garlic products sales. We are all in debt for the benefits the research of this wonderful natural panacea has brought.

Certainly we must act responsibly and ingest the best quality food we can, exercise and, when possible, supplement our diets with products like Preven-CA, Barleygreen, Kyolic or another of the excellent products now available. But remember that even good things can be taken to extremes. What is dangerous about exaggeration is intolerance; let's not kill ourselves in the process of improving our health. Do not convert your nutrition into a religion, eat well, have fun exercising and enjoy life, neither too little nor too much.

Chapter $\boxed{7}$

Between Heaven and Earth

> Thirty centuries have been required to know its structure.
> It would take an eternity to know something of its soul.
> Not more than an instant is needed to kill it.
>
> **Voltaire**

Man Confronts Creation

For centuries, man survived nature's harshness with no technological advances. 3000 years ago, man was freed from the countless obstacles in his way by learning to manipulate his environment, all of this without the help of medical science. Yet, disease brought with it the need for a cure. In primitive cultures, there existed procedures in which all kinds of spirits were evoked with the hope of healing the sick.

Little by little, those with acute perception took note of the fact that the body responded to certain elements like water, herbs, seeds, etc. They observed that certain foods produced specific effects. So began the art of medicine. In its beginning, medicine took advantage of the herbarium available to diverse, ancient cultures. The Aztecs were outstanding in the world of their day, relying on more than 1000 registered medical plants. The Greeks learned to distinguish the symptoms of specific diseases, observing that the diseases were subject to natural laws and that they generally responded to certain elements. In our day, we can ratify the discoveries of their cures when we use home remedies. The body calls out for what it needs. When we have the flu, our body asks for herbal teas, broth (Jewish penicillin), and rest. Less money and lives would be lost if we would just listen to our bodies!

According to the modern-scientific-uncommon-sense medical establishment, some "waco" doctors in Paris, France, are treating "terminal" patients (to me there are only terminal illnesses) in the most outrageous, inhumane way. In this clinic of torture, the patients are "forced" to fast as long as their condition will permit. When they can't take it any longer, they are seated, with eyes blindfolded, in front of a table with organic and natural foods. My god!

With the guidance of their olfactory sense alone, they, the tortured, choose what their bodies are hungry and thirsty for. The patients instinctively choose the foods that contain nutrients lacking in their organism (the true cause of their illness). The ones who have emotional and mental disorders will pick foods rich in neuro-transmitters like thiamin and niacin. Those with arthritis, will stay away from hyper-allergenic foods and eat the ones with anti-inflammatory properties like garlic; cancer patients invariably will choose foods with immune empowering capabilities like broccoli and sprouts as well as those that have anti-tumor qualities like seeds (Amygdalin, phytochemicals and antioxidants) and garlic. The results are surprising to the doctors (not to me) because many will go home healthy and sane.

Instinct is one of the mechanisms God has given us for the preservation of our health. We could call it organic wisdom. Unfortunately, doctors and their progressive science have separated us from these instincts, this wisdom. But that's not all medical science has not considered. It has also bypassed the emotional impact and the spiritual needs that illness brings with it. Who, in his right mind, does not look inside and seek divine intervention when arthritis, diabetes, multiple sclerosis or cancer strike? Believers pray harder and atheists suddenly doubt the nonexistence of God!

Modern Christian believers that follow spiritual guidance in many aspects of their lives also have placed their fear on germs and, though we believe in the supernatural power of God, put our trust in antibiotics and dangerous medical treatments. In the past 100 years, we have lost touch with ourselves and our creator. It pains me, but physicians have much to do with the social attitude that all must have scientific proof. Doctors have set out to destroy the faith of their patients. Have I not mentioned plenty of scientific reports in this book to give weight to my points of view? Why? Because I am (as well as you -my dear reader) accustomed to, and conditioned to prove my case. However, let's not forget the highly effective technique initiated by the Nazis, "If we repeat a lie often enough, it will be taken for the truth." By this method the huge medical industry has, for almost two centuries, been persuading us to think that it has the answers -there must be scientific explanation- otherwise, it's all in your mind! Yes, precisely what matters is in your mind, only doctors have not exploited its power. Scientists have dedicated years to study and have come to understand the functioning of the marvelous human body. This I don't criticize. Today, we are at the threshold of having, through the study of genes, the blueprint of the body, the genoma, the body's atlas. Yet, we have not advanced very much in the war against disease.

What has happened is that as we (doctors) continue on our quest to be the best qualified and sophisticated body mechanics, we completely push aside the mind and spirit of our patients. There is no doubt in my mind that our failures spring from this fact. It cannot be blamed on technology or academic pursuit but on the abandonment of the philosophical principles of medicine. We have cast aside basic premises like, "First do no harm," and, "Thou shalt love thy neighbor (patient) as thyself." If we would respect these principles and apply them in our daily practice, doctors would be more conscientious. We would feel more compassion for our fellow man and we would be more effective if we intervened less. We have in truth blinded ourselves to reality. In our quest for proof, we have relegated the spiritual factor. J.M. Cano, a Spanish song writer, says it well, "Between heaven and earth there is something, and that something is I." This "I" is the mind and spirit within our body which seek God, especially in trying times.

God: Creator or Created ?

Philosophy affirms that belief in God is a weakness. We need God so much that we invented Him or create Him. The agnostics say that it is easier for a person to believe in God or to become very religious when overcome by illness because we want a miracle. But believers affirm that God is our creator and is able to do what man can't do. In time of pain, we can draw near to seek his grace and help. "God is our refuge and strength, a very present help in time of trouble" (Psalms 46:1). For those of us who accept the divinity of a creator, there is access to spiritual blessing. I have seen that those who hold genuine love for God and sustain a close relationship with him, confront disease with greater strength. There are intrinsic biochemical mechanisms that are set in motion by our state of courage and spiritual strength.

The Mind And Body Communicate With Each Other

We have already seen how environmental, nutritional and genetic factors can contribute to diseases like cancer. However, depression, suffering, and anger are even more fearsome enemies.

Positive or negative attitudes act as messages from our mind, conscious or unconscious, capable of engaging biochemical processes in our organism that directly affect the state of alert of our immune system. Body functions, from an insignificant muscle twitch to the amount of white cells circulating, all are dependent on our state of mind. We will perform better, whether in tennis or chess, when we are rested and happy. We will better overcome infections if we are happy and rested. These mechanisms now supported by scientific research, are far from being understood, but we know they are activated or blocked by biochemical messages, probably through enzymes or hormones like the endorphins.

Mixed Messages

One day a patient that had been given a death sentence in New York came to see me. He was told to settle his affairs and get ready to die in a few weeks. The patient, an affluent lawyer, desperate because he couldn't find anyone to offer him any help in the United States, decided to take a plane and travel to Mexico. Why, I asked, would a scholar choose to come to a retrograde country, of all places Tijuana, the new Sodom, to seek help from a quack? He replied, "Because you are the only one who offers me some ray of hope." This man was willing to cross frontiers, not only geographical but cultural, to demonstrate that he was committed to regain his *body's* health. "What is that you have in your shirt pocket?" I asked him. "It's a pack of cigarettes," he replied. I said, "Sir, you have lung cancer. Don't you think it would be a good idea to stop smoking?" His response was, "Yes, I definitely know that is what I ought to do but I haven't been able to stop."

Here is an example of a clear discrepancy of messages. On the one hand, the patient is saying to his body, "I am so interested in *you* that I am willing to travel to Mexico. I have been given up on but I will try alternative medicine. I want to go on living." On the other hand, by refusing to quit smoking, the patient is saying to his body, "My commitment does not include doing away with the pleasure of smoking, even though cigarettes are killing *you*." The healing process requires that the patient be 100% committed to getting well.

Getting well... what does it take? There are many factors involved, yes, but it all boils down to the impact each one of those factors has on the immune system. Because of its importance I feel it's necessary that you understand, even superficially (don't think that doctors do profoundly!), the means your body counts on to maintain health. Come with me through the abbreviated tour.

The Immune System

The master work of creation is the human being, but with all the splendor and greatness that God gave us, our survival is still very fragile. In this world, plagued by invisible aggressors, the importance of defense mechanisms looms large. Although our body relies on some natural barriers like the skin, nasal hair, mucous secretions, and inflammatory processes, the bulk of the defense task falls on the immune system. The moment a microorganism enters our body, an elaborate and extremely intricate attack is launched. The capillaries dilate like flexible tunnels to admit an army of defenders. These defenders are called leukocytes. Like all truly efficient lines of defense, the immune system fixes an attack with a strategy that is divided initially into two types of responses, the nonspecific and the specific.

The Nonspecific Immune Response

This type of response is the main system of defense for newborns until they develop antibodies. However, the nonspecific immune response never ceases to be useful and necessary. Some tribes of white corpuscles called **monocytes** and **phagocytes** are charged with attacking any invader never before encountered. From the monocytes, the **macrophages** are derived. Present in almost all organic tissue, they have the mission, like a *pac-man*, of surrounding and disintegrating undesirable cells. From the phagocytes the **microphages** are derived. These are divided into two sections, the **neutrophils** and the **eosinophils**. The neutrophils are a large army and are in charge of disintegrating invading bacteria. The eosinophils, a more select group, target foreign substances like cells covered by antibodies and allergens.

The Specific Immune Responses

This one develops after birth as a response to microorganisms and their toxins. A gigantic task that can only be given to the awesome **lymphocytes**. They are so called because they are produced by lymphatic ganglia. A fourth of all white cells are lymphocytes and are divided in there branches, **T-cells**, **B-cells**, and **killer cells** which are distributed strategically according to specific needs throughout the body. The T-cells are **cytotoxic**, in other words, they intoxicate the invaders through chemical warfare. This is such an important line of defense that 80% of the lymphocytes are T-cells. The B-cell lymphocytes (15%) are more specialized, they produce the mighty **immunoglobulins**, which are exceedingly important antibodies that maintain the memory of specific chemical substances which will destroy a specific invader, a process which is called **humoral immunity**. The **killer cells** are the SWAT team of the lymphocytes (5%). They charge with brut force invaders or aberrant cells like cancer or cells infected with a virus.

The Immune System In Action

So then, the leukocytes in all their branches are the members
of the assault troops when outside invaders put us in danger.
Invisible, loaded with weapons, slippery fighters, they float
around the cells, good and bad, like a Mexican taxi driver on a
busy boulevard, to confront pathogenic microorganisms face
to face. Seen through a microscope, the lymphocytes look
like over-easy eggs sprinkled with ground pepper. Each "little
dot of pepper" is a deadly chemical weapon. The neutrophils
in the bloodstream inflate themselves like balloons before
they attack. The microphages seem to just lay around, buried
among the tissues, but spring into life when there is an attack. The neutrophils, armed with proteins and nonspecific
chemical agents, do the job of common soldiers, attacking
the enemy with brute force and a numerical advantage. The
lymphocytes, with membranes protected in an imposing way,
arrive with the heavy artillery, like combat tanks. Their strategy may vary. While some lymphocytes float in the blood
and attack any foreign microorganism that travels along, others plant themselves in vital organs and pursue any invader
who may have gotten past the first line of defense. Still other
lymphocytes corral the invaders in the lymph nodes which
serve as execution chambers.

When the battle is over, the neutrophils gather up cellular refuse and perform a vital cleanup job. Because pathogens can camouflage themselves with chemical barriers made up of cellular refuse, cytoplasmic seepage, coagulating agents and destroyed membranes, the clean up crews are led by the antibodies, which guide the lymphocytes to the camouflaged pathogens. Although the antibodies are 1000 times smaller than bacteria, they attach themselves to their enemy like "banderillas" attached to a bull in a bullfight, weakening and neutralizing its irregular forms in preparation for the definitive attack by the "matador," the leukocytes. In healthy periods, 25 billion leukocytes circulate freely in the bloodstream and another 25 billion rest on the walls of the blood vessels and other tissues. When an infection appears, billions of reserves leap into the bloodstream from the reserves in the bone marrow. The blood can quickly mobilize up to ten times the normal number of white cells, which is the way doctors measure the seriousness of an infection. The higher the number of leukocytes in the blood, the greater the degree of virulence. The first time an agent invades our bodies, one of the circulating lymphocytes (B-cells) comes in contact with this pathogen, memorizes its shape and size and dashes to the nearest lymph node where this lymphocyte turns into a chemical factory, transferring the recently acquired information to thousands of other lymphocytes which also turn into factories of antibodies. In a few hours the body can count on billions of antibodies, specifically designed to kill the new invaders. Once the lymph nodes produce an antibody, the formula remains stored permanently so that when the aggression is again present, the response can be immediate.

The antibodies are the highest expressions of **specific** immunity. An antibody protects our organism from a single affliction. For example, the antibody against the measles virus has no effect on the smallpox virus.

The timing of the immune response determines success more than the act itself. The time our body needs to organize its defenses is crucial. It is here where the antibiotics shine, destroying millions of bacteria, giving the body time to arrange a defense. But an antibiotic never kills all the germs. Even if it kills all but one, that lone microbe can immediately reproduce itself in industrial quantities. Only the immune system does away with 100% of the invaders. Today we can understand this concept by looking at AIDS victims. It doesn't matter how many pounds of antibiotics we administer. The infection continues to run its course because the immune system has been paralyzed. Sometimes the invaders have a shape so complicated that the defense mechanisms can't decipher it. The plagues were devastating examples of this.

Even with all these setbacks, we can't deny that the human race has survived all these centuries, thanks to the immune system. You may not believe or be aware of it, but this complex, sophisticated defender of the human race is deeply affected by our attitudes, emotions and spiritual fortitude.

George Lilans, a Boston psychiatrist, followed 200 Harvard graduates for 30 years during which he correlated data from medical examinations and psychological tests. He found a clear connection between unhappiness and disease or death. Lilans concluded that good mental health promotes physical health. Who is responsible? ...The immune system.

Most of my patients can relate to a stressful situation in the past that they feel triggered their cancer. But how can you measure the impact our emotions have on the immune system? The following is a scale created by Dr. Thomas H. Holmes and Dr. Reji of the University of Washington Medical School which measures each stress situation with a point system.

Death of a spouse	100	Heavier responsibilities	29
Divorce	73	Children leaving home	29
Separation	65	Wife starting work	26
Imprisonment	63	Start or finish of classes	26
Death of a family member	63	Change of residence	25
Sickness or accident	53	Change of personal habits	24
Marriage	50	Problems with boss	23
Stopping work	47	Change of work hours	20
Reconciliation in marriage	45	Change of neighborhood	20
Retirement procedures	45	Change of school	20
Family illness	44	Change of recreation	19
Pregnancy	40	Change of church	19
Sexual Problems	39	Change of social activities	18
A new person in the family	39	Small mortgage	18
Personal readjustment	39	Change of sleeping habits	16
Financial adjustment	38	Separation from family	15
Family Discussions	35	Change of diet	15
Mortgages above $25,000	31	Planning a vacation	13
Debt foreclosure	30	Christmas activities	12

Holmes and his collaborators were able to predict illnesses on the basis of this scale. Almost half (49%) of the people who had accumulated 300 points in a twelve month period developed some critical illness while only 9% of those who accumulated less than 200 points in the same period fell ill. This experiment irrefutably establishes the impact that accumulated stress can have on our body. There are people who have a large capacity for managing stress so they are less susceptible to falling ill. On the other side, losing one's job at 25 years of age is not the same as losing it at 50, nor is it the same thing to end a marriage by common consent than to end it in the midst of a furious battle. It seems important to me that happy, positive events as well as sad or problematic ones can cause stress. Getting married, for example, can mean joining oneself to a beloved person and therefore it is a happy event. Even so, it implies an adaptation that requires effort on the part of both parties. Either way, bear in mind that our emotions determine the response of our immune system. Why do some, under similar stressful situations, fall ill and others don't? Barring the inconvenient exceptions, it all depends on *how* we react in the face of adversity or success.

Hopelessness, Pessimism, Frustration and Unhappiness

Arnold Huchnaker wrote, "Depression is a partial surrender to death and it seems that cancer is desperation at the cellular level." We are under emotional pressure constantly. There are crises and wars everywhere. How can we avoid the stress which anguish, fear and depression cause? The actions and reactions of our body are responses to, more than anything else, the attitude with which we confront the events, problems, challenges, experiences, memories and expectations of our lives. Researchers are just discovering how depression, pessimism, excitement, and optimism directly and physically affect the reactions and capabilities of our immune system. Again late, Galen, in the second century, had already affirmed that depressed men or women more easily fell prey to cancer than those of a more sanguine temperament.

There is evidence that housewives who feel useless contract cancer with 54% more frequency than the general population and 157% higher incidence than women who work. Wives and mothers who feel they make a substantial contribution, because they are an irreplaceable team member in the family, have a lower incidence of cancer. These statistics were published by Dr. William Morton of the University of Oregon. What an awesome correlation between frustration and dissatisfaction and the crippling of the body's system of defense. For example, divorced persons have the highest index of cardiovascular disease, pneumonia, high blood pressure, cancer and, even though you may doubt it, a higher incidence of fatal accidents (camouflaged suicides?). Did you notice that divorce causes more stress than imprisonment? The amount of couples splitting for irreconcilable differences is staggering.

It's creating a society of depressed, resentful adults and of children who hate themselves, because "they were the cause of the divorce," or hate their parents for abandonment. It shouldn't surprise us that *Time* magazine in its April 25, 1994 issue stated that, "The history of hate in the family is one of the primary factors which determines the risk, the risk of contracting cancer, the most devastating plague of the 20th century." The power of negative emotions, like depression, unhappiness and hate, is enormous. History revolves around their dominance, especially hate. It leads to war, destruction and death. There is only one other emotion comparable, but more powerful: Love. "For love is stronger than death," says the Bible in Songs of Solomon 8:6.

Love, Hope And Optimism

Humans are obsessed with the negative. Have you ever seen a TV news broadcaster that gives only good news? I heard some lunatic tried that and promptly went bankrupt. Loads of research demonstrate that stress is bad and that, of all the contributing causes of disease, at least 75% are because of it. Well, common sense would say that there is little need to investigate the contrary, that happy and satisfied people seldom get sick. But our health professionals are not in the habit of taking for granted the obvious.

The happy person is not the one who has only good things happen to him or her, but that person who keeps a positive attitude even in adverse conditions. Habakkuk, in the midst of good times, cried out, "Although the fig tree shall not blossom, neither shall fruit be in the vines, the labor of the olive shall fail and the fields shall yield no meat, the flocks shall be cut off from the fold and there shall be no herd in the stalls. Yet, I will rejoice in the Lord. I will joy in the God of my salvation. The Lord God is my strength and he will make my feet like hind's feet and he will make me to walk upon mine high places" (Habakkuk 3:17-19). This Biblical passage shows that Habakkuk was ready and willing to keep a positive outlook, giving thanks even if his fate would turn for the worst.

The concept that we are children of the Almighty God that literally worries about our problems is mythical for most. God is a concept, not a being, much less a "person" of action. Jesus said, "What father among you, if your son asks for bread, will give him a stone? Or if he asks for fish, in the place of fish, will he give him a serpent? If you then being evil know how to give good gifts to your children, how much more will your Heavenly Father give the Holy Spirit to them that ask him?" (Luke 11:11-13). If science convinces you that this is unreasonable, you cannot take advantage of the benefits faith provides.

If you instead embrace the offer and earnestly reasonably put your trust in God, your perceptions about life and its problems begin to shift. The reason why the action of God is often suffocated and strangulated is because we don't dare to acknowledge what we are in Christ. "But in all these things we are more than conquerors through him who loved us." (Romans 8:37). If in the face of a need we confess that the Lord is our shepherd, we will lack nothing. (Psalm 23). He is our supplier. Our success will be measured by our confession and the tenacity with which we cling to that confession. Remember, "What I confess is what I possess." If I confess Jesus as my Lord, I possess salvation. If I confess that "The love of God has been shared abroad in our hearts," (Romans 5:5) I possess the capacity to love each human being.

You have to be very careful with dualism. If you confess that you have faith in the word of God, but you doubt that he can deal with your disease, you are guilty of dualism. A positive confession will free us from the burdens which have been thrown on us. If we profess sickness, incompetence, sadness, poverty, helplessness, resentment or hatred, should we expect health, strength, happiness, abundance, faith, pardon and love?

I'm not proposing that strong faith bearers do or should not have struggles -we do- but our faith helps us handle things with a different reaffirming and "solution-ability" perspective. The Bible says, "To those who love the Lord, all things are for their own good." (Romans 8:28). Surely it is not easy to act very positively when problems arise, but we can take help from someone who is greater. It is God who works with us, in us and for us. When we ask from God, it is valid to ask for what is beyond our power to understand, what is above our reach or what we have not been able to do. Let's cultivate the habit of thinking big and we will learn to use words that will allow God to make us conquerors. Let's not say that we can't when God has said He can.

The diplomat and famous first lady of the United States, Eleanor Roosevelt, said, "No one can hurt you without your consent." This profound assertion clearly states that we determine our situation. In Mexico, a culture rich in faith, we say that, "Evil comes so that blessings will follow." So many spend their whole lifetime **waiting** for the ephemeral "blessings to follow." What benefit can come of my mother dying when I'm 10? Where is the advantage of being diagnosed with cancer? Abraham Lincoln said, "Things may come to those who wait, but only the things left by those who hustle."

I have no definitive answer, but an example can help. A patient of mine diagnosed with testicular cancer at 38, a deadly tumor, said, "Having cancer was the best thing that could have happened to me." I gave him the "excuse me?" look. "You see doc," he continued, "I took life for granted; money came easy and life came easy. Now that I'm facing death I appreciate my wife, whom I hurt so much, my abandoned children, I even appreciate a rainy day!" It is attitude not circumstances that helps us understand that "all things are for our own good." Those who anchor themselves to these wise proverbs, the optimism they embrace will show them a way to keep life from embittering them. Critics will say that this is just brainwashing. Doctors prefer to not stain their professionalism with such empirical and foolish popular beliefs. God forbid!

So, the affluent, successful, intelligent (well, let's call them, higher-than-average-IQ) conservative, rational Harvard professionals that choose to be frustrated, desperate and sad and full of hatred (because that makes more sense) are falling prey like flies to heart attacks while the equally affluent, successful, intelligent (whatever…), not so conservative and not so rational Harvard graduates that are "foolish" enough to be optimistic dreamers, happy and loving live longer and better, according to Dr. Vaillont's not so empirical findings. Can this be why the born comedians in general live longer than the rest of the population? "A merry heart does good like a medicine." (Proverbs 17:22).

Love

A most revealing work has been done in Israel by Jack Medoli and Yuri Goldbert. The two researchers studied 10,000 men with high risk conditions like angina pectoris, anxiety, high cholesterol, and irregular heartbeat - all the requirements for a fatal cardiovascular condition. They determined, through psychological testing which would develop a heart attack and which would not. After all was said and done, the ones who had the highest incidence of heart attacks were the ones who answered "NO" to the question "Does your wife show you love?"

Insurance companies have discovered that men who are dismissed in the morning with a kiss from their wives are better clients because they will have fewer car accidents and will on the average live five years longer, as reported by Leo Buscaglia in *Living, Loving and Learning.* If it wasn't because insurance companies are in the business of evaluating risk to increase their revenue, I wouldn't believe it either, but there it is, simple and romantically scientific! These revolutionary findings of the 20th century were well known centuries ago to the Hebrew people. "Rejoice with the wife of thy youth." (Proverbs 5:18). "He who finds a wife finds a good thing." (Proverbs 18:22).

"Wisdom rests in the heart of him who has understanding but it is not found in the fool." (Proverbs 14:33). I find no other way to explain why doctors do not take advantage of this powerful knowledge in their daily practice.

Although love research is in its infancy, studies are beginning to confirm its positive effects. The Menneger Foundation of Topeka, Kansas, found that people who were in love have lower levels of lactic acid in the bloodstream, which causes them to feel less tired and that they have higher levels of endorphins, which cause them to feel more euphoric and less sensitive to pain. Their white corpuscles respond better to infection and they catch fewer colds.

It is not surprising then to know that the essence of the Biblical message is love, immortally described by St. Paul in one of his letters to the church in Corinth:

> Though I speak with the tongues of men and of angels and have not love, I am a sounding brass or a tinkling cymbal and though I have the gift of prophecy and understand all mysteries and all knowledge. And though I have all faith so as to remove mountains and have not love, I am nothing. And though I bestow all my goods to feed the poor and though I give my body to be burned and have not love, it profits me nothing. Love is long suffering and kind. Love does not envy. Love does not vaunt itself, is not puffed up. It does not behave itself in an unseemly manner, seeks not her own, is not easily provoked and thinks no evil. It does not rejoice in iniquity but rejoices in the truth, bears all things, believes all things, hopes all things, endures all things. Love never fails but where there are prophecies, they shall fail. Where there are tongues, they shall cease. Where there is knowledge, it shall vanish away. And now abides faith, hope, love, these three, but the greatest of these is love."
>
> *1Corinthians 13*

In 1982, Harvard psychologists, David McClelland and Carol Tishnit, discovered that even films about love increase human levels of immunoglobulin-A in saliva, the first line of defense against colds and other viral diseases. Although this immunological improvement lasted less than an hour, it could have been prolonged by having the subjects think about moments in their lives when someone loved them. If we love, we are happy and those around us make up a part of our positive world and don't wear down our defenses.

Struggle And The Power Of The Mind

Stories of two of my patients exemplify the dramatic power that love and hope provide to one and the destructiveness of lack of love and hopelessness to the other. A young woman, 19 years of age, came in to see me. Her doctors had given up hope and diagnosed her with cancer of the small intestine. A course of chemotherapy offered no positive results. Under these conditions, her prognosis was death within three to six months. This girl was a member of her country's team which in eight months would participate in the Olympic games in Montreal. She said she had come to me because she did not accept the prognosis of her doctors and that she would under no circumstances stay out of the competition. She began her treatment with a lot of faith and discipline. The results were indeed amazing. In all sincerity, our results with patients with this type of tumor are pessimistic but the determination and tenacity of this girl stimulated her defenses so powerfully that they destroyed her tumor. In reality, the treatment only served as an emotional reinforcement. All she needed was somebody to give her hope, someone who would show interest and love. To date, this patient is alive and healthy.

On the other side of the coin is a 48 year old woman with breast cancer who came to us after having been treated surgically. They had removed her left breast. Her cancer had been complicated by metastasis in the bones and lungs. Conventional therapies had failed and her doctors had sent her home to die. At the start of our treatment, one could faintly see the remains of her former beauty. She looked as though she had been in a concentration camp, skeletal and bald. All of this was the result of an aggressive and unsuccessful treatment with chemotherapy. Little by little she began to improve. Her hair grew back, she gained weight and the beauty of her face began to reappear. In six months, she was a new person. Although surgical mutilation had dealt her a painful blow, she had overcome it. Once her husband saw that she was strong enough he decided to ask her for divorce. Under any circumstances this is devastating event, it was augmented by the fact that she interpreted it as a rejection of her mutilated body. In three weeks, she experienced an explosion of tumors. Although she came back to see me, she confessed that the loss of her husband's love represented the worst kind of rejection and life had lost all meaning. No human power was able to change her perspective. Her immune system gave up and the tumors took advantage of the open doors and killed her.

Love is so important and powerful that Christ summarized nine commandments into one, the golden rule, "Love your neighbor as you love yourself." Yes! "All we need is love…" sang John Lennon, but why is there so little of it? My brother-in-law, Joel Ordaz, an independent minister, believes that precisely because we love our neighbors as *we love ourselves* there's so many problems in our world!

Contradicting perspective; but lct's examine how we love ourselves. We love junk food, alcoholic beverages and smoking. Love is never having to exercise. Our love affair with quarreling, fighting and hating is at an all time high. Your neighbor certainly doesn't need this kind of love.

Self-esteem in every culture is vital to the preservation of good health, both physical and mental. Narcissists just love their looks but people who love or esteem themselves accept the fact that we are imperfect beings. Once you and your defects are comfortable with each other, you are more likely to be happy in this world. Those who are at peace with themselves and others enjoy a longer and better life. This love of self includes accepting responsibility for the health of your body, soul and spirit; this is the "yourself" love your neighbor needs. But even with our imperfections, love is still the answer.

Abusive Authority

Love for the patient in the medical field has long ago been exchanged for the passion in the quest for pathogens. Feelings, emotions, fears and expectations are ridiculed. When doctors face a desperate patient, instead of hope, they deliver a scientific *honest* verdict, "You had better settle your personal affairs. According to the statistics, you will die in a few months." Desperation turns to absolute hopelessness. After all, the sentence was given by an authority. It's true we have earned it by spending many years of study and sacrifice, but this authority is reinforced because the patient grants it to us. I mean, not many professionals have the authority to undress you in their offices! What the doctor says is law. This authority would be useful if applied to changing our patient's destructive habits. But, in view of the awful results of our illustrious scientific intervention, a patient would do better to disobey the doctor. For example, if an oncologist tells a patient that he only "has three months," he will be anxiously waiting to fall dead on that day. "I can't let my excellent and qualified doctor down!" Too many patients are still conditioned to obey such terrible orders. Indeed, with unkind words, "not more than an instant is needed to kill," Voltaire, again, knew much about medical practices.

The Deciding Vote

Probably the most important difference of the practice of alternative doctors is their focus on the overall well-being of the patient rather than the conventional aim at the destruction of the disease. In the case of cancer, conventional therapies have lost time squandering money in the search for the cause of cancer when, as we have seen throughout this book, it is perfectly well known that there is not a cause for cancer but a combination of causes. Each one of us reacts in a different way and the response to treatments is varied, none-the-less there is no variability in the inefficiency of orthodox therapies. Beyond this, we have forgotten to take human behavior into account. Fortunately, more and more people have become aware of the noxious effects of modern medicine and are seeking non-aggressive natural treatments. Proof of this is found in data provided by the *New England Medical Journal.* In 1992, people made 425 million visits to doctors offering alternative therapies and 388 million to allopathic doctors. On the other side, allopathic therapies cost 60 times more. Assuredly, the cost in lives was also a lot higher.

The hurting are making a statement, they need no more of it. Our trust in democracy has lost value. Most people vote without the conviction that it matters, but when we vote with our money, we are casting a powerful "yes" vote. This kind of vote is effective and brings about change. By making more visits to alternative doctors, people are promoting the kind of attention they want -medical practice that focuses on the whole patient's needs rather than on disease. The fact that allopathic doctors are being hit in the pocketbook will promote change. Kizer Permanente has been forced to accept alternative therapies like acupuncture and nutrition in order to maintain their leading slot in the HMO business. Unfortunately, they, as well as most doctors, have not demonstrated true interest in changing their philosophy. Moreover, they haven't shown even the slightest interest in re-evaluating or changing the proven ineffective conventional therapies. The alternative medical movement is far from perfect, but it has had an eye-opening effect on patients, doctors and health authorities that is going to be impossible to suffocate.

Spiritual Ties

Essentially we are designed to be a unified creature but the pace of modern life doesn't leave room to cultivate a whole and balanced life: body, mind and spirit. We cannot be divided. Those that give exclusive importance to the body but neglect intellect and the spirit are failing to practice adequate medicine. Many famous psychologists, Jung for example, recommend the cultivating of the spirit to help preserve health. Some do not refer precisely to the relationship of the human being to God, but rather to a relationship to beauty through art. Yet, I have found all through my medical practice that the cultivation of the spirit is to be understood as the relationship of a man with God. The spirit is that part of our being that allows us to communicate with God. It is what allows hopeless human beings to recuperate the essence of life in a supernatural way, to discover life as one has never experienced it before.

The patients who "throw in the towel" almost always do so because of the negative attitudes of their doctors, when they say "There is nothing more to do." But our hearts tell us that, "Hope dies last." In my experience, there is dignity in the struggle, in fighting the invincible foe. Even when hope fails, if you fight, there is a feeling of satisfaction from having given the enemy a tough fight. Life, to a great degree is at our disposal. We have control over our decision to fight or fold. We can't change the past but we can choose the present and decide our future wearing the armor of hope and not anguish.

Every person who has spiritual ties, independent of religious beliefs, lives longer and better; but the great advantage of Christianity is that it is founded on love. "For God so loved the world that he gave his only begotten son that whosoever believes in him should not perish but have everlasting life." (John 3:16). This manifestation of the love of God to mankind is what enables us to love ourselves and others. It also is the foundation of hope that whatever we do is not in vain, that we are going to a special eternal place where there will be no more sorrow or pain.

Resources: Scarcity Versus Abundance.

o see the human person as a trinity -body, mind, and spirit- and to treat him as such in the practice of medicine is something I learned from my father. When I chat with my patients, I make sure that they leave with useful hope that can help them confront their condition. As I broach the subject of stress, which is very common, I define it as a deficit of resources needed to resolve a problem. This is a simple definition but adequate. If you have enough money to pay the rent, there is no stress, but anxiety reigns when you hear the footsteps of the landlord and you have to give him an excuse!

Success against any adversity requires that you recognize and face the obstacles first, and secondly, the positive, optimistic utilization of the resources at hand. It is an illusion to *hope* for a life without problems, to ask God for help is not. At the OASIS of Hope Hospital, patients get bodily resources, yes. But they are presented with the opportunity to receive Christ as their Savior because He represents an inexhaustible fountain of resources. This is why patients with strong spiritual ties with God can better face disease. They can deal with the initial rage, frustration and despair that all people experience when they find out they are suffering from a disease. They trust in God and they have hope. They keep a positive spiritual attitude because they fortify themselves with prayer and by reading His Word. The patient who knows he is saved through the merits of Christ does not fear death because he knows where he is going. Many cast aside these concepts as simplistic but they forget that all human beings in every culture and religion know intuitively that we are spiritually eternal. As a doctor, I am concerned about giving my patients good quality for their fleeting physical life, but shouldn't I also be concerned about their eternal life? We often defeat disease but sometimes it defeats us. One day, sooner or later, we will cross from this terminal life to another which has no end. We don't want any of our patients to depart without knowing that living in Christ is the best life, now and forever.

Epilogue

Where there is no wise counsel, the people perish but in the multitude of counselors, there is safety.

King Solomon

Governmental authorities continue to defend present health care structures in spite of irrefutable evidence of their failure. All my findings have led me to the conclusion that orthodox medicine and its science are a failure. Time, money and human resources have been squandered in the search for the cause of many chronic degenerative diseases for more than a century. Humanity has paid this dogmatic scientific experiment with too many lives already. Searching for a cause is futile, the aggressors are nothing, the *soil*, "our internal environment," is everything. Drugs have failed because each person responds in a different way to them and in many cases the therapy is worse than the disease. The mechanization and dehumanization of the practice of medicine have dismantled the human being and managed to convert physicians into mechanics of the body disregarding the mind and the spirit.

I recently participated in a conference on alternative treatments in Washington, D.C. One of the scientists, upon discussing reports published about some natural "remedies," said that he kept himself away from such publications. With a raised eyebrow and a disdainful look similar to that we make when we see a dirty animal approaching, he commented that such reports were printed in magazines of little prestige without the scrutiny of other scientists with experience in the field. The strongest and most competent criticism leveled against alternative medicine is that there is no data published in "peer reviewed" journals -journals that require evaluation by experts in the field, such as the *New England Journal of Medicine*, *Journal of the American Medical Association* and others. On the rare occasions when research on alternative methods are presented for publication, they are rejected because they don't fulfill all the strict and dogmatic rigidity of the scientific method established for the protection of academic integrity.

I am in no way implying that alternative medicine should be exempt from these requisites, but the rules of the game were established with prejudice. For instance, natural substances that are not under the umbrella of economic patent protection, are at a disadvantage because there are no grants to support their investigation. A new agency to evaluate alternative therapies has been established. Bravo! Their annual budget of 2 million dollars is not even sufficient for payroll. The NCI gets at least 1.5 billion dollars a year and with the last 30 billion they've come up empty handed. Sometimes I visualize these ministers of science, guardians of academia and its statutes solemnly exercising their responsibility to accept or reject the arduous labor of researchers, like those judges who make the accused sweat it out until they read the verdict. The fallibility of these judges is made more obvious by the ominous impact and consequences that their honorable decisions make on society. They permit publications that benefit only the economically involved and avoid the publication of others that are soundly scientific, by different criteria yes, but that offer practical and efficacious alternatives. I never tire of reiterating the accomplishments of critical medicine since I have to boast about something in this now, semi-sublime profession. If it weren't for that, it would be difficult to call myself a doctor. But I will not stop exposing how useless the scientific method has been (and those who apply them) in the treatment of chronic diseases.

Thousands of gallons of ink have been wasted on "peer reviewed" publications authenticated by experts in hundreds of prestigious journals regarding "approved" orthodox therapies. In spite of all this "publisistic" enthusiasm, the incident of new cases of cancer and of those who die from this disease continues to explode. In the last four decades, chemotherapy research has made the headlines of the majority of medical journals with all the academic fanfare, applause, prizes and the solemn acceptance of the experts with authority on the subject. The researchers are happy, their universities and institutes have obtained more money for their impressive advances, the industry is bulging with profits and the patients are dying. The only conclusion that can be drawn is that their (pseudo) therapeutic value borders on the criminal. My professional pride cries out for the academic recognition of the establishment, that the authorities of the oncological branch would give me their blessing. My conscience as a physician nevertheless demands that I offer to my patients sufficient resources so that he or she can decide which route to follow in their struggle to recover health.

In spite of all the propaganda being made by advanced technology in the health services and the accomplishments in critical care medicine, people have become conscious of the atrocious results of modern dehumanized medicine. For the first time in the history of the USA scientific medical era, doctors have received a bad grade and have lost about 30% of their business to alternative medicine as published by *New England Journal of Medicine*. Most of the patients (80%) that went to seek help from the "infra doctors" got what they were looking for, but paid 60 times less than those who received treatment from the overqualified physicians. Democracy leaves a great deal to be desired, but patients are overwhelmingly voting with their consultation money to have alternative medicine. The medical industry has to accept that alternative medicine will become the preferred option for the population. Not even the might of the establishment can stop the power of this life preserving paradigm shift

Tendentious Information

After a lecture on these matters, a friend and colleague, Dr. Ismael Cosio, a dedicated gynecologist felt offended because of the severe criticism I leveled against present medical practice. He refuted my severe position against the establishment, criticizing the information I quoted from medical, scientific and environmental literature as tendentious.

Before I answer this valid criticism, let me say that I recognize that in no other profession will you find more people dedicated to the service of humanity. All of us have worked hard. I remember 72 hour long shifts, attending patients in the operating rooms and hospital wards when I was simultaneously completely asleep, yet awake; totally worn out, yet tireless; sad, yet motivated. It's true that we have a "call" to do it but what motivates us more is the example given by teachers and fellow students in hospitals, schools and the consultation rooms. Yes, doctors in general are there to serve, even in countries where they are excessively remunerated.

But our professional life and dedication is tightly controlled by rules, regulations and laws provided by the establishment. Our intervention is dictated by published research unavoidably attached to economic strings.

This compromised information in my opinion is tendentious. Tendentious information directs with bias toward a certain thought pattern or way of thinking. It necessarily has a component of gain which almost invariably is economic. For example, Coca-Cola always says that Pepsi Cola is not as good. Medical practice is governed by a scientific cannon, strictly conforming to and controlled by the system, the establishment I have so roundly criticized. We get these norms from information published in books and magazines which set forth the criteria (tendencies) to which we must adhere. We treat our patients with protocols, procedures and products dictated by the industry and government. They control everything because they have an irrefutable conflict of interest.

Let's take for instance, the President's Cancer Panel of the United States (established in 1971), which is a group assigned to supervise, control and promote cancer research in institutions such as the Memorial Sloan Kettering, the American Cancer Society (ACS), the National Health Institutes, especially the National Cancer Institute and others. Its first director was the famous New York lawyer, Veno

Schmidt, a banker and investment capitalist of Wall Street who gave an enormous push for cancer chemotherapy research. Although totally useless, these toxic drugs are increasingly recommended by doctors. The cancer industry today is an extremely profitable enterprise. The value of the stock of the pharmaceutical laboratories that produce "chemo," thanks to Schmidt's intervention, has mushroomed incredibly and, by the way, the aforementioned individual held a large number of shares in those laboratories which brought him an enormous personal fortune. He was in office "only" 10 years. The following ten years belonged to Armand Hammer, president of Occidental Petroleum, one of the worst environmental offenders. This monstrous enterprise is responsible for the infamous contamination of "Love Canal" (Chapter 2) with highly carcinogenic agents which, conveniently, has never been properly investigated.

Interestingly, from 1971 to 1991, the pillars of anticancer research were in the hands of people with tremendous conflicts of interest, to put it mildly. One profits while promoting useless and deadly anti-tumor drugs and the other, a representative (and protector) of the main producers of carcinogens.

The productivity of the cancer industry (in all its modalities) in the United States is calculated at 10 billion dollars annually. In chemotherapy alone, 515 million were spent in

1985. In 1990, the amount rose to 1.2 billion. In 1995, the take stood at 2½ billion, and at the turn of the century will touch 5.6 billion (all in U.S. dollars). Naturally, the interested parties will defend "the market" tooth and nail, sparing no resources.

Medicine in general is an enormous business. In the USA, it is calculated at one trillion dollars annually. Although in Mexico and other less rich countries, the numbers aren't as exorbitant, we are manipulated by the same tendentious information which we wouldn't dare question for fear of being accused of heresy by our northern teachers. Doctors are at the front line of action in the medical industry, governed and manipulated by "scientific" information which without doubt fulfills the function of keeping us in line with a perfectly oiled sociopolitical and economic establishment.

But the image of the medical corps is going downhill by gigantic steps. While we were once the very symbol of dedication and sacrifice in the search for health, the general public has now relegated us to a place over there with the suspicious gills of lawyers, used car salesmen and politicians. What does my tendentious denunciatory information get for us? Surely those of us dedicated to alternatives could be economically favored by the paradigm shift. I hope so. But although natural products are on the rise, gains are ridiculously small in comparison to those of the pharmaceutical industry. The consumption of organic products has multiplied in spite of the negative "scientific" information that questions their added nutritional value. What governmental authorities and scientists cannot deny is the incredible positive impact this mode of farming would have on our environment. Doctors that promote natural therapies and companies that produce nutritional supplements should be applauded; not ostracized and persecuted. From my tendentious point of view, I will list some of the consequences of this anti-establishment information and important impact it could have on the health of the population.

- Increase prevention awareness.
- Enormous savings in medical costs.
- Research for and by the people; not for the industry.
- Halt to unnecessary medical intervention.
- Increase utilization of natural effective therapies.
- Dramatic fall of iatrogenic deaths.
- Better utilization of hospital installations and medical services for the management of true emergencies.
- Total care approach, body, mind and spirit for all patients.
- Respect for the laws of nature.
- Improve the image of our medical establishment.
- A better world for our children.

The Enemies Of Health

Many critics of the establishment take things very much "to heart," accusing government, industrialists and doctors of perpetrating a "conspiracy against humanity." That is giving them too much credit. To qualify as a conspiracy, there must be philosophical ideals for which people will risk all. I see the position of the establishment as a very worldly one - money. Any change of the establishment means a very substantial loss of income for them. In the 80s and 90s particularly, the supreme value around which all human activity revolves has been money. The objective of industry, professions and business, has lost the meaning of mission. The single goal of generating profits has alienated them all. It's the same with the publishing industry. The goal is not to print books to disseminate information but to earn money. Private physicians are more concerned about how many consultations they will have and how much cash they will take in than about the health of their patients. The food industry doesn't concern itself with nutrition. Even worse, it floods the market with substances that are poisonous to the organism, and all to generate profits.

James Patterson and Peter Kem, in their book *The Day America Told The Truth*, have named the 80s the "decade of greed." The majority of people in the United States say that "greed isn't so bad as long as it doesn't make you fat." Greed being understood to mean the passion to be excessively rich.

I'm sure the reader will agree with me that this name can still apply to the 90s. The new trend in greed is that it has invaded areas considered before untouchable and immoral, such as doctors profiting from human suffering. I do not believe that money has ever been evil, but greed always has. Man's true evil nature becomes most visible when he takes away from others so that he can have more for himself.

The interesting thing is that the people (in a large part) responsible for our miserable state of health have become rich without taking money from us. We have voluntarily given it to them when we consume products that destroy our environment, foods that make us sick, services and medical procedures that are dangerous and medicines that are highly toxic. Who are the true enemies of health? We will quickly point our accusing index to the political and scientific authorities. In principle I agree, the most responsible ones are those who are in a position to approve and disapprove what the public consumes. It took a lot of digging, but no major difficulties to gather all the inflammatory information regarding this book. Imagine how much classified research there must be in the archives not open to the public? How much money have industrialists spent to bury certain information, in falsified research or with "bribes" to get rid of it? Our lives depend on such Establishment!

When the acceptance of failure is unavoidable, the medical industry conveniently shields itself with establishment data that frees them from all blame and responsibility. The treatments have been *proven* to work and it can't be helped if genetic factors, habits and abilities (or lack of them) of patients are the cause of the failure. In other words, sick people don't know how to choose their parents. They smoke, drink and eat too much, and to top it off, they don't even know how to respond to the therapies prescribed by their doctors. Yes, the establishment would have us believe it's all the fault of those ungrateful patients.

In the wake of the third millennium I encourage myself and fellow doctors to take responsibility for our own actions and embrace dreams not so impossible any more, thanks to pioneers like Dr. Ernesto Contreras Sr., and stop blaming patients, industrialists and politicians. Like Don Quixote, let's fight for the triumph of good, justice, beauty, and love. Love for our patients and our profession. Doctors should become health specialists. The disease oriented practices will be crushed as patients seek alternatives. Taking the "narrow road" the Bible recommends has inconveniences but the rewards are immeasurable. The physician that wants to survive in the 21st century will have to take care of the whole patient - body, mind and spirit - and love his patient the way he loves himself. We must practice medicine in harmony with our sacred oath. Our mission is commitment to the life and well-being of our patients; not staying within the favor of our teachers and authorities who have degraded our philanthropic profession.

While the authorities have not and will not apply the death penalty that Hippocrates recommended for violating his oath, the world medical corps that continues to practice dehumanized medicine will surely perish. Praise God!

Lastly, the most important enemies of our health are ourselves. We certainly sin much by omission because authorities and doctors adulterate or hide important data but, in this era of information overload, excuses are futile; every day it becomes harder to make fools of ourselves. Do you really believe that the doctors are responsible for your health? Take matters in your own hands. Let's not leave our most highly valued possession, our health, in the hands of unscrupulous people who are only interested in their pocketbook.

Please don't think that the advice I give here is something I have completely mastered. However, I hope and pray this information helps you, as it has helped me personally, and professionally to take responsibility for my health and my surroundings. There is nothing easier than giving advice. We hate to ask for it since we usually already know the answer, and when we do ask, we hope to hear justification for our actions rather than chastising. Walter Benjamin, a German philosopher, said that, "Advice intermit with action is knowledge." I have reproduced here the advice of multiple authors to give you "safety," as quoted earlier (Proverbs 11:13).

The goals initially will seem difficult and far away but every journey begins with the first step.

I hope the recommendations found herein will be practical and reachable. Let me close by urging politicians to take care of people and our land, the industrialists to stop polluting it, the medical profession to fulfill its mission and me and you to be responsible for our health. Let's take a vow to provide for our own bodies, minds and spirits, all available resources for the enjoyment of better health. Let's leave a moral legacy and a better world for our children. I bless you, your family, and the world's population with health in the 21st century.

Bobbie & Barry Teitler
303 Oakridge Ct.
Bellevue, Ne. 68005
1-402-291-8302

Andrea & Dave Iverson
PO Box 32924
Juneau, AK 99803
907-789-5754

(Dave's 50th Birthday)
Sept 10th

Capt Peters' Birthday
Aug 10th

Sunday Jan 17th   Flight to Antigua

Monday   Antigua

Tuesday   St. Barths

Wednesday   Nevis

Thursday   Iles de Santes

Friday   Dominica

Saturday   Martinique

Sunday   St. Lucia

Monday   Bequia

Tuesday   Mayreau

Wednesday   Palm Island

Thursday   Carriacou

Friday   Granada

Saturday   Flight home   Boo

SOURCES AND RECOMENDED READING

Chapter 1. A Race Against Time.

Albestrand, Kaj et al. *Life extenders and memory boosters,* Health Quest Publications, Reno, Nevada, 1993, 348 pp.

Atkins, Robert C. *Health revolution. How complementary medicine can extend your life,* Houghton Miflin Company, Boston, 1988, 422 pp.

Beasley, Joseph D. *The betrayal of health. The impact of nutrition, environment, and lifestyle on illness in America,* Times Books, 1991, 274 pp.

Burton, Kathy and Gary Yanker. *Walking medicine. The lifetime guide to preventive & therapeutic exercise walking programs,* McGraw-Hill Publishing Company, New York, 1990, 480 pp.

Darrach, Brad. *"The war on aging",* Life, October 1992, pp. 32-43.

Lafee, Scott. *"Science finds clues to old age in basic biology"* The San Diego Union Tribune, March 1, 1995, section E, pp. 1, and 3.

Schmidt, Karen F. *"Old no more"* U. S. News & World Report, March 8, 1993, pp. 66-73

Zoglin, Richard. *"Good night, George. George Burns 1896-1996".* Time, March 18, 1996, p. 99.

SOURCES AND RECOMENDED READING

Chapter 2. Back To The Future

Babini, José. *Historia de la Medicina.*, Gedisa, 1a. edición, Barcelona, 1980, 204   pp.

Beasley, Joseph D. *The betrayal of health. The impact of nutrition, environment, and lifestyle on   illness in America,* Times Books, 1991, 274 pp.

Comisión Metropolitana para la Prevención y Control de la Contaminación Ambiental del Valle de México. *Avances sobre la evaluación y modernización del Programa "Hoy no circula",*   México, 1994.

Comisión Nacional de Derechos Humanos. *Contaminación atmósferica en México, sus causas y efectos,* México, 1992.

Conferencia de las Naciones Unidas sobre el Medio Ambiente y el Desarrollo. *Declaración de   Río sobre el medio ambiente y el desarrollo.*

French, Hilary F. *"Making environmental treaties work",* Scientific American, December 1994, pp.   62-65.

García, Delfín. "Veneno en la piel", *Muy interesante,* año XII, no. 1, pp. 40-46.

Lacouture, Genevieve Francois. *Relacion entre los seres vivos y su ambiente,* Editorial Trillas,   México, 1983.

LaRue, Steve. Chemicals preying on sexual function" *The San Diego Union   Tribune,* August 31, 1994, section E, pp. 1 and 12.

Leff, Enrique. *Medio ambiente y desarrollo en México,* Universidad Nacional Autónoma de México, México, 1990.

Leutwyler, Kristin. *"Deciphering the breast cancer gene",* Scientific American, December 1994, pp. 18-19.

Programa Integral Contra la Contamination Atmospheric dell Vale de Mexico, Mexico, 1990.

Quadric de la Tore, Gabriella. *Desarrollo sustentable. Hacia una política ambiental,* UNAM, Coordinación de Humanidades México, México, 1993 176 pp..

Sachs, Ignacy. *Desarrollo sin destrucción,* El Colegio de México, México, 1982.

Secretaria de Educación Pública. *Introducción a la educación y salud ambiental,* México, 1987.

Sharpe, Richard M. y Niels E. Skakkebaek, "Are estrogens involved in falling sperm counts and disorders of the male reproductive tract?" *Lancet,* vol. 341, May 29, 1993, pp. 1392-1395.

Suárez, Luis. *La contaminación,* Fondo de Cultura Económica, México, 1974.

Suzuki, David y Peter Knudtson. *Génetica. Conflictos entre la ingeniería y los valores humanos,* Traducción de Josée Sanmartin y Marga Vicedo, Editorial Tecnos, Madrid, 1991.

Thompson, James y Margaret Thompson. *Genética médica.* Salvat Editores, 1983, 401 pp.

SOURCES AND RECOMENDED READING

Chapter 3. Hunger Is Vicious

Avila Curiel, Abelardo. *Hambre, desnutrición y sociedad. La investigación epidemiológica de la desnutrición en México,* Editorial Universidad de Guadalajara. Guadalajara, Jalisco. México, 1990, 175 pp.

Banco Internacional de Reconstrucción y Fometo/Banco Mundial. *La pobreza y el hambre. Temas y opiniones sobre la seguridad alimentaria en los países en desarrollo,* Washington D.C., 1986, 79 pp.

Beasley, Joseph D. *The betrayal of health. The impact of nutrition, environment, and lifestyle on illness in America (*Times Books, 1991, 274 pp.

Encyclopedia Britannica, fifteenth edition, 1985

Grunwald, Lisa. "Do I look fat to you?" Life, February 1995, 58-74.

Kradjian, Robert M. "Milk. The natural thing?" *Newlife,* New York, November /December 1994, pp. 31-37.

Solórzano del Río. Héctor. "Efectos colaterales por consumo excesivo del azúcar refinada", *El Occidental,* Guadalajara, Jalisco, México, July 31, 1994, Section E, p 3.

Suzuki, David y Peter Knudtson. *Genética. Conflictos entre la ingeniería genética y los valores humanos,* traducción de José Sanmartín y Marga Vicedo, Editorial Tecnos, Madrid, 1991.

SOURCES AND RECOMENDED READING

Chapter 4, "111"

American Cancer Society, *Cancer facts & figures - 1996, Atlanta, 1996, 28 pp.*

Anonymous, "El método científico pervertido, *Muy interesante, año XI, no. e, México, 1994, pp. 6-8.*

Anonymous, "Errar es de sabios", *Muy interesante,* año XI, no. 3, México, 1994. pp. 10-13.

Anonymous. "Fraudes, mentiras y líos científicos. Los piratas del laboratorio", *Muy interesante,* año XI, no. 3, pp. 14-17.

Anonymous. "The chemo's Berlin wall crumbles" *Cancer chronicles,* December, 1990, p. 4.

Bailar III. John C. and Elaine M. Smith. "Progress against cancer?", *New England Journal of Medicine (NEJM),* vol. 314, no. 19, May 8, 1986, pp. 1226-1232.

Balkany, Thomas. "Why unconventional medicine", NEJM, vol. 238, no. 4, Jan 28, 1993, p. 282.

Beardsley, Tim. "A war not won", *Scientific American,* January, 1994, pp. 130-138.

Begley, Sharon. "Beyond vitamins". *Newsweek,* April 25, 1994, pp. 44-46.

Begley, Sharon and Daniel Glick. "The estrogen complex, *Newsweek,* March 21, 1994.

Bier, Jerry. "Shark cartilage a cancer cure?" *The Fresno Bee,* November 28, 1993, section A, pp. 1 and 20.

Bogdanich, Walt. *The great white lie. How America's hospitals betray our trust and endanger our lives,* Simon & Schuster, New York. 1991, 320 pp.

Castro, Janice. "Condition: Critical. Millions of Americans have no medical coverage, and costs are out of control. here are 10 ways to fix what ails us" *Time,* November 25, 1991. pp. 34-42.

Chung, Connie. "Eye to eye with Connie Chung", television program, CBS, February 2, 1995.

Clancy, Yankelovich and Shulman. "The new era of alternative therapies", *Time,* November 4, 1991.

Clark, Cheryl. "Natural born Killer", *The San Diego Union Tribune,* August 31, 1994, section E, pp. 1 and 3.

Dowling, Claudia Glenn. "Fighting back breast cancer" *Life,* May 1994, pp. 78-88.

Eisenberg el al, "Unconventional medicine in the United states. Prevalence, costs, and patterns of use" *NEJM,* vol. 328, no. 4, January 28, 1993, pp. 246-252.

Friend, Tim. "Unbiased information hard to find", *USA Today,* July 27, 1994.

Grolier Electronic Publishing, 1992

Hamburguer, Jean. *La miel y la cicuta. Sobre la diversidad de los seres vivientes,*

SOURCES AND RECOMENDED READING

Chapter 4, "111"

traducción del Francés por Juan José Utrilla, Fondo de Cultura Económica, México, 1989, 149 pp.

Ingelfinger, F.J. "Laetrilomania", *NEJM,* vol. 296, no. 20, May 19, 1977, pp. 1167.

Inlander, Charles, Lowell S. Levn and Ed Weiner. *Medicine on trail. The appalling story of medical ineptitude and the arrogance that overlooks it.* Pantheon Books. new York, 1988, 394 pp.

Kurtycs, Anna. "Por las alcantarillas de París", *El Occidental,* Guadalajara, Jalisco, México, Julio 31, 1994, sección E, p. 1

Lemonick Michael. "the killers. New viruses and drug-resistant bacteria are reversing human victories over infectious disease" *Time,* September 12, 1994, pp. 62-69.

Lisa, P. Joseph. *The assault on medical freedom,* Hampton Road Publishing Company, 1994, 384 pp.

Marantz, Paul. "Beta carotene, vitamin E, and lung cancer", *NEJM,* vol. 331, no. 9, September 1, 1994, pp. 611.

Mendelsohn, Robert S. *Confessions of a medical heretic,* Warner Books, New York, 1979, 297 pp.

Michaelmore, Peter. "Un médico con casta" *Selecciones,* Abril 1993, pp. 117-122.

Mullins, Eustace, *Murder by injection,* The National Council of Medical Research, 1988 361 pp.

Murray, Raymond and Arthur Rubel, "Physicians and healers - Unwitting partners in health care", *NEJM,* vol. 326, no. 1, January 2,. 1992, pp. 61-64.

Nash, Madeleine, "Stopping cancer in its tracks", *Time,* April 25, 1994, pp. 54-61.

Podolsky, Doug and Rita Rubin. "Heal thyself", *US News & World Report,* November 22, 1993, pp. 64-76.

Ruiz, Carmen. "Cuando los médicos matan", *Contenido,* February 1995. pp. 101 - 107.

Salaman, Maureen. *The cancer answer. . . nutrition,* Statford Publishing, Menlo Park, California, 1984, 309 pp.

Shilts, Randy. *And the band played on,* Penguin Books, 1988, 646 pp.

Suskind, Patrick, *El perfume. Historia de un asesino,* traduccion del Alemán por Pilar Giralt Golina, Seix Barral-Editorial Planeta Mexicana, México, 1994 [1985}, 237 pp.

Toufexis, Anastasia. "The new scoop on vitamins", *Time,* April 6, 1992, pp. 54-58

Vintró, Eulalia. *Hipocrates y la nosología hipocrática,* Ediciones Ariel, Barcelona, 1972.

Werth, Barry. *The billion dollar molecule. One company's quest for the perfect drug,* Simon and Schuster, New York, 1994, 455 pp.

SOURCES AND RECOMENDED READING

Chapter 5. The Possible Dream

Carper, Jean. "Alimentos que ayudan a prevenir el cáncer. *Selecciones del Reader's Digest,* Abril, 1994, pp. 69-73.

Coperías, Enrique M. "Alimentos contra el cáncer. La cesta de la vida", *Muy interesante,* año XII, no. 2, pp. 18-24.

Kim, Peter and James Patterson. *The day America told the truth,* Plume, new York, 1992 {1991}, 270 pp.

SOURCES AND RECOMENDED READING

Chapter 6. Neither Too Little Nor Too Much

AIM International. *The concept of the healthy cell,* Nampa, Idaho, no date, 125 pp.

Albestrand, Kaj el al. *Life extenders and memory boosters,* Health Quest Publications, Reno, Nevada, 1993, 348 pp.

Anonymous, "Back to butter?", *University of California at Berkely Wellness Letter.* vol. 10. no 11. August 1994, p. 1.

Asmead, Dewayne H. *Conversations on chelation and mineral nutrition,* Keats Publishing, Inc. New Cannan, Connecticut, 1989, 240 pp.

Beck, Melinda. "An epidemic of obesity", *Newsweek,* August 1, 1994, pp. 62-63.

Burton, Kathy and Gary Yanker. *Walking medicine. The lifetime guide to preventive & therapeutic exercisewalking programs.,* McGraw-Hill Publishing Company, New York, 1990, 480 pp.

Cardona, Gloria, Esperanza Rascón y Raúl Paz. *La salud por los alimentos,* Arbol Editorial, México, 1988, 170 pp.

Coperías, Enrique M. "Alimentos contra el cáncer. La cesta de la vida", *Muy interesante,* año XII, no. 2, pp. 18-24.

Cott, Allan. *Ayuno: La dieta máxima,* traducción del Inglés por René Cárdenas Barrios, Editorial Diana, México, 1994 {1997}, 165 pp.

Cowley, Geoffrey, "Are supplements still worth taking?", *Newsweek,* April 25, 1994, pp. 47-48.

Diamond, Harvey y Marilyn Diamond. *La antidieta. Unos principios claros sobre cómo alimenrarnos; lo importante no es lo que se come, sino como y cuando se come,* Ediciones Urano, 1986, 245 pp.

Hendler, Sheldon S. *The doctor's vitamin and mineral encyclopedia,* Simon & Schuster, New York, 1990.

Garduño, Roberto. "Abajo de niveles mínimos de nutrición, 24 millones", *La Jornada,* Junio 19, 1994, p. 21

Mosqueira, Guillermo F. *La salud y los alimentos,* Publicaciones Mundonuevo, México, 1986, 243 pp.

Murray, Mary. "Can these pills make you live longer?", *Reader's Digest,* September 1994, pp. 19-26.

Orozco García, Octavio. "Leche: mal alimento para los Mexicanos", *El Occidental,* Guadalajara, Jalisco, México, July 31, 1994, sección E, p. 3.

Passwater, Richard A. *Cancer and its nutritional therapies,* Keats Publishing, Inc., 1978, 256 pp.

Prasad, Kedar N. *Vitamins in cancer prevention and treatment. A practical guide,* Healing Arts Press, Rochester, Vermont, 1994

SOURCES AND RECOMENDED READING

Chapter 6. Neither Too Little Nor Too Much

Rodwell, William, Sue. *manual práctico de nutrición,* Editorial Pax, México, 1987 {1973}, 262 pp.

Swope, Dr. Mary Ruth, *Green Leaves of Barley,* Swope Enterprises, Inc.

Thompson, James and Margaret Thompson. *Genética médica,* Salvat Editores, 1983, 401 pp.

Whang, Sang. *Reverse aging. Not science fiction but a scientific fact ,* Sang Wang, Miami, Florida, 1990. 123 pp.

Wright, Jonathan V. *Dr. Wright's book of nutritional therapy. Real-life lessons in medicine without drugs,* Rodale Press, Pennsylvania, 1979, 519 pp.

SOURCES AND RECOMENDED READING

Chapter 7, Between Heaven And Earth

Angell, Marcia. "Disease as a refection of the psyche", *New England Journal of Medicine (NEJM)*, vol. 312, no. 24, June 13, 199

Burns, David, *Sentirse bein. Una nuva fórmula contra las depresiones,* Mexico, Paidós, 1991, {980}, 424 pp.

Cousins, Norman, *Anatomy of an illness. As perceived by the patient,* Bantam Books, New York, 1989 {1979}, 173 pp.

Frankl, Viktor E. *El hombre en busca de sentido.* Editorial Herder, Barcelona, 1994 {1979}, 132 pp.

Gossett, Don and E. W. Kenyon. *The power of positive confession of God's work,* Kenyon Gospel Publishing Society, Washington, 1978 {1977}, 95 pp.

Seigel, Bernie S. *Love, Medicine and miracles. Lessons learned about self-healing from a surgeon's experience with exceptional patients,* Harper & Row Publishers, New York, 1986, 244 pp.

Simonton, Carl O., Stephanie Mathews-Simonton and James L. Creighton. *Getting well again,* Bantam Books, New York, 1992 {1978}, 287 pp.

SOURCES AND RECOMENDED READING

Epilogue

Beardsley, Tim "A war not won", *Scientific American,* January 1994, pp. 130-138.

Kim, Peter y James Patterson. *The day America told the truth,* Plume, New York, 1992 {1991}, 270 pp.

Eisenberg et al. "Unconventional medicine in the States. Prevalence, costs and patterns of use", NEJM, vol. 328, no. 4, January 28, 1993, pp. 246-252

Ultra Health Int.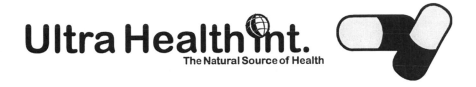
The Natural Source of Health

4360 Border Village Road
Suite 203
San Ysidro, CA 92173

Tel. (619) 428-0930
Fax. (428) 428-0994

Also Available

To You, My Beloved Patient

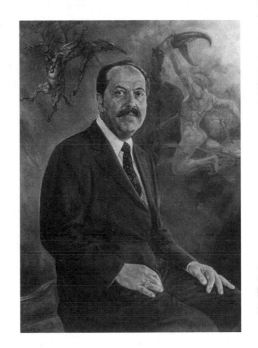

The autobiography of Ernesto Contreras, Sr. is the heartwarming and incredible story of how one highly recognized and respected doctor was ostracized and labeled a quack by the same medical establishment that once claimed him to be one of its finest. Committed to finding the most effective and compassionate treatments, Dr. Contreras Sr. pioneered alternative therapies and the holistic approach.

Through the exile from the orthodox world of medicine and threat of incarceration, he never lost sight of why he did the things he did. It was always for his beloved patients.

VIDEOS

- *OASIS HOSPITAL's Institutional Video, Body, Mind and Spirit*
- *What The Bible Says About Disease.*
  Ernesto Contreras, Sr., MD
- *Sing Along and Love & Laughter*
  Ernesto Contreras, Sr., MD and Shary Oden
- *The Disease and Host Relationship*
  Ernesto Contreras, Sr., MD

Send Orders to:

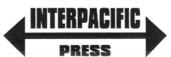

INTERPACIFIC
PRESS

PO BOX 7597
CHULA VISTA, CA 91912

To order by phone, call (619) 428-0930, weekdays, 9-5 Pacific time.
We accept VISA and MASTERCARD, or send a check or money order
payable to Interpacific Press. 1-800-950-6505

KEYNOTE SPEAKER

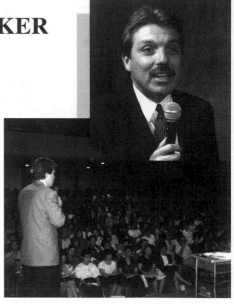

FRANCISCO CONTRERAS, MD, is accomplishing his mission to improve the quality of the physical, mental and spiritual lives of the world by taking his message of hope to conventions and meetings, as well as by appearing on television and radio talk shows. He has presented at conferences throughout the USA, Canada, Mexico, Japan, Korea, Australia, Spain and Slovakia. He personally oversees more than 600 patients with cancer every year at the world renown Oasis of Hope Hospital but his conviction to have a global impact takes him around the world to at least 70 engagements each year.

Curriculum Vitae
Specialty:
Oncological Surgery, University of Vienna, Austria - 1983
Alternative Therapies, Oasis of Hope Hospital, Tijuana, Mexico - 1978
Current Position:
General Director, Oasis of Hope Hospital.
Conferences/Events:
12ᵗʰ International Tumor Markers Conference, New York; National Health Federation;
Cancer Control Society; AIM International; Cornerstone Television and others.

" *This dynamic and motivating health specialist has given our organization a powerful impulse. He is one of the most requested speakers by our distributors (who total more than 70,000 worldwide) for our local area training seminars."*

Ron Price
Executive Vice President, AIM International

"*Dr. Francisco Contreras continues to pack them in year after year at NHF conventions. He is heartwarming, informative and entertaining."*

Maureen Kennedy Salaman
Fifteen-Year President of the
National Health Federation

If you have an important meeting, and wish to present profound health-related truths and dispel the myths of modern medicine, please write to:
INTERPACIFIC PRESS
PO BOX 7597
CHULA VISTA, CA 91912
or call: **1-800-950-6505**
We will be happy to send you a press kit and discuss arrangements. It is best to plan at least six months in advance.

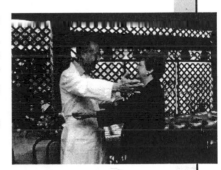
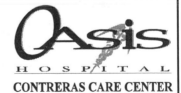

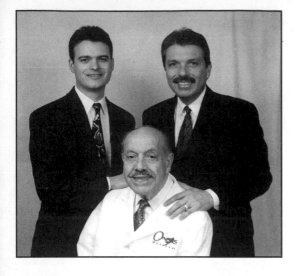

Three generations of Contreras are working together for one mission – To provide services and an environment designed to improve the quality of the physical, mental and spiritual lives of people around the world. It is not the fact that the Contreras's Oasis of Hope Hospital is a modern fully equipped medical/surgical facility with world-class specialists that draws people to them. People seek their care for more important reasons. The Contreras love their patients as themselves and they offer the most effective and compassionate therapies that are uplifting to the body, mind and spirit. They are recognized for their unique blend of competence, commitment and compassion. With all of the love, hospitality and expert care patients and companions receive from the staff at the hospital, many have been inspired to call the Contreras Center – *An Oasis of Hope*.

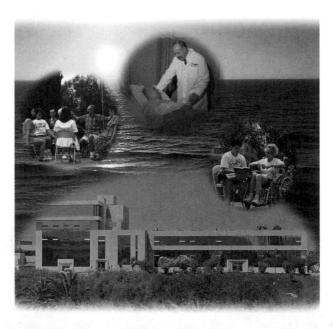